The Journey Begins

August 27, 2007

What a dream! I had tea with Jesus!

OK-my dream was the doorbell rang so I answered it. I was home alone, and being alone is pretty rare so this dream was going well already. Jesus was standing on my front stoop. He smiled at me; what beautiful eyes. I almost didn't say anything because I was memorized for a moment. My polite training from my mom kicked in, and I said to Jesus, "Please come into our home, Jesus."

Jesus said, "Thank you, Patty. I have a message to give you."

Wow, Jesus and I are on first name basis - I don't remember being taught at CCD class what to do if Jesus comes knocking at your door, so I did what I thought was best: I offered Him a cup of tea.

I made us tea and we sat down at the dining room table. I was in awe that Jesus was in my house. We made small talk while I sipped my tea - I don't remember that part. Jesus then stood up; tea untouched, and said He needed to go.

He looked at me, took my hands, and said,"You will be given results that you will believe will destroy your world as you know it. This is not going to happen. You are not alone. You will always have Me walking beside you, helping you find God's grace to get through what seem to be dark days with the tools of love, support, and courage. You will need to look, and sometimes you will need to look hard. Remember, I will never leave you." He hugged me and left.

I woke up, startled. It took me awhile to remember that I was in my bed and everyone was sleeping. My mind was trying to wrap itself around the dream. It was the most realistic dream I have ever had. I could still feel Jesus' hug. Since I couldn't fall back asleep, I went downstairs to get a

4

glass of water. When I reached the dining room table, I almost screamed. There on the table were two tea cups- one empty and one full.

I dropped to my knees, shaking. I prayed to God to give me the strength that I now knew I was going to need for the rest of my life. I had a doctor's appointment later that day where I would receive the results of my biopsy test. I knew I was going to be told that I have cancer: Breast Cancer.

I don't let fear run my life. I have no way of knowing what tomorrow brings, but I know I have the power of today. With the help of God's grace, family, and friends, I have been able to get through the darkest of days (diagnosed to stage 4 and the loss of my sister-in-law to breast cancer) with grace and eyes wide open to try and find the positives in all situations.

I want to thank you for your love, support and most of all, prayers. Jesus is right; I am not alone.

Let the Blogging Begin...

The cocktails for my treatments:
Here are the chemo drugs I will be taking for the 8 treatments. I get one mixture for 4 weeks and another for the last 4 weeks - but I don't know what comes first.
Cyclophosphamide
Adriamycin
Taxol
Herceptin - this will be given to me pending my Fish test from my biopsy. I haven't heard what the results are, and to be honest I am not quite sure what it means. If it comes back with numbers that require this drug then I will ask questions.

I guess I will go get the day started. If anyone has good recommendations of some funny stories, I could use ideas. I really enjoy reading and I am thinking about taking the Amtrak downtown for my treatments. I think the ride is a little over an hour. I am not sure of what it is like during treatment. I have heard about getting a DVD player for movies, but I think I would rather read.

I have been told that by the third treatment that I will be bald. I am not sure what to think about that right now. It seems like that will be the smallest of the problems I am facing.

Well I went with two friends and got a wig. I thought it would be easy to get, but it was a lot harder than I'd thought. It was a good thing I didn't go alone because I probably wouldn't have gotten one. I also picked up some turbans and add-on bangs - that was very cool. I had thought about taking pictures but am very glad I forgot the camera. I am not someone who can wear long hair at all. No one ever needs to see that look on me. Have a wonderful day - and thanks again for the prayers. I know that they are working because I am getting out of the house, and I am not letting this take any more from me. GI Jane is getting ready to show her strength and to kick some ass!!!!

Getting ready to become Bald and Beautiful,

Posted Aug 25, 2007 9:45pm

Another new one for me: For those who don't know, my brother, Jimee, is getting married in November and - here is the big news of the day - I already have the outfit purchased and hanging in my closet. I still need shoes (what woman doesn't need shoes?) but I don't think I have EVER got an outfit this early for anything, including my own wedding. I am not a big shopper, but it is nice to have that done. Also, if my skin is yellow and weird looking in November, I will know that at one time I was a hot mama in this outfit and will be again.

I am a bit nervous about the start of chemo on Friday. I am having a port put in but it won't be able to be used until the second treatment. During one of my tests they took blood out, mixed it with something so toxic that if we drank it we would be in the ER, and then put it back in me. My vein collapsed and they had to find another one. Please pray for strong veins for Friday - they can be wimpy after that because the port will carry the load for the rest of the treatments.

I am going to be styling during chemo. I was given two Spirit-Sister outfits to wear. They are pink and very soft. No ugly hospital gowns for me.

Of course, Becca will be telling me to wear the wig with the outfit, going to bed, picking her up from school, getting the mail, drinking my tea and wherever else she deems a wig is necessary. She does not want a bald mother - she has been telling me this for the last two days. She is better off having a bald mom then a long hair blonde (on me!!). Trust me on this because there will be no pictures!

On that note I shall say good-night. Talk to you later.

7

Well the Fish test came back and it's negative - which is positive. I asked what would have happened if the results were positive (always trying to learn something new every day). I would have had to go every three weeks for a year for a chemo treatment. I am glad I waited to ask that question. I might have lost some beauty sleep on that one.

In case I didn't update you, my port placement was rescheduled for Friday and the chemo is still on for Friday. Rob and the girls, Ryan (brother) and Sue (sister-in-law) (for those who didn't know my BABY brother was married a couple of years ago), will be hanging out with me. If anyone else wants to send a picture, I will bring you to chemo with me. Please include your family. I have been getting emails from friends of long ago and it is so wonderful.

Any pictures that I get before the 14th of September will be singing Happy 40th (silently, of course, because even in Harry Potter books the photos didn't make noise).

Take care and have a great day!!

I just wanted to send a quick note to say thanks again for all the love and support. I haven't gotten back to all the Marquette and AT@T people who have sent emails, but you have all brought me smiles.

My last day of "normal" life is to go to the Lincoln Park Zoo. Hopefully my nephew, Aidan, and Sharon (sister-in-law) will be able to join us-and enjoy this picture perfect day in Chicago.

Tomorrow at 9:30am the port is surgically placed; then 1:30pm is chemo. I am not sure how I will feel about this new journey that has been thrust upon me, but I will try to post something this weekend.

The kids (Raney 9; Becca 7) start school on September 4th @ 8:00am.

Please remember that even though I might not respond quickly to your emails, I am grateful for them and I will respond at some point.

Love to all.

Posted Sep 2, 2007 4:27am

Well, I can't hide the fact that I am up at an ungodly hour but, for the future, I was given a prescription that is to help with the inability to sleep. I think that I am supposed to wait until Tuesday to start taking it. I didn't have my brother, Jimee, in the room when the nurse was telling Rob and me about when to take what, and I can't remember. (Such pressure for you, huh, Jimee?) I will call the hot-line tomorrow to ask.

We never made it to the zoo on Thursday but did visit with Sharon. (Aidan slept through most of the visit. He was awake for a few minutes.)

That night Raney and Rob went to the pre-season Chicago Bears game. Becca and I joined my dad, Jimee, Kristin (future sister- in- law), and Katy for dinner at a great Cuban place, Cafe 28, on Irving - if you ever have a chance to go, I highly recommend it. After dinner, we went to Margie's - a great ice-cream place. Jimee was sent a Shrek hat and I wore it to the ice cream place. Becca was quite embarrassed. My Shrek ears were never straight. My message is too long, I have to split it into two so, to be continued...

Posted Sep 2, 2007 4:28am

The next morning was calm. I was on no-solid food after 3:30am and a no-liquids diet after 7:30am. My port was placed in on time and that was (and still is) tender. They told me that could be sore for up to two weeks. That is one of the problems for sleeping; my left breast hurts to lie on and now the right side hurts too - but it all will be done soon. Something is going to go: the boob or the port. My family won't want a 'Crabby Patty' because of lack of sleep (my nickname from my children because of SpongeBob SquarePants).

9

I knew I should have never let the sweeties watch TV. I even have my youngest accusing me of being crabby if I haven't had my tea yet.

Chemo: We had a wait before we got a room (we were on the 21st floor with an awesome view of Lake Michigan) but once we got in, the port was usable (so my vote is to keep the port and get rid of the breast that started this whole journey). If memory serves me, I think it was about 2 hours once I was hooked up. We finished in time for Chicago rush hour traffic so Ryan, Sue, Niki, Jimee, Rob, Raney, Becca, and I went to Gino's for pizza and pasta.

The ride home was a bit uncomfortable because of the port (maybe the port just lost its vote; so hard to know what to do) but we made it.

Saturday my sister-in-law and her family came up to help with school clothes shopping. Diane is also making some meals to freeze.

I was told that the effects from the chemo are cumulative, so right now I still feel fine; getting a little bit of a sick feeling in the stomach but nothing too bad at the moment.

OK, I should probably have typed this in the beginning, but one of my prescriptions is to help with memory - I don't think I have started that one either - so please no grading my grammar, spelling or typing! Thank you.

One more thing, and then I will try to get back to sleep before everyone wakes up. My friend Ann, who is a doctor, came over to give me a shot to boost my white blood cells. I just want to thank her again. The needle was not a big deal but the medicine was a bit painful. I probably would have yanked it out with the first drop. I am such a baby sometimes.

Last thing: GI Jane's (aka GI Patty's) haircutting party is still on for September 12th. I was told my hair will start to fall out on the 14th. What a wonderful fortieth birthday present— going bald. I am sure that is on everyone's birthday list. Now that is the one thing that I remembered from the nurse: I will be losing my hair soon.

I am enjoying the quietness of the house, and since it has been a long time since I was bald, I may be choosing what I want to remember. I was a very cute bald baby so I hope that this is not going to be as hard as I am imagining.

Thanks again for your thoughts and prayers. I need the tumor to shrink or stay the same size or I go in for surgery the next day. And my white blood cells need to be at the right number or they delay chemo a week. One down and 7 to go!! We are on the right path and thanks for being on it with me!!!

Posted Sep 4, 2007 6:15am

Good Morning! For those friends who are not aware, today is the first day of school and Raney and Becca are dressed. This will be the only time this year that they are dressed 2 hours before school starts. I can't believe that they are up. Last night was a disaster trying to get them to sleep. I had taken a pill to help with nausea, which also causes drowsiness. Raney and Becca kept calling for me and wanting to sleep with me so I just went downstairs to sleep. I thought for sure I would still be pulling Becca out of bed at 10:00am this morning, but the excitement of school is far greater than the lack of sleep. Hopefully they will be on the schedule of getting up with no problem for at least the first week.

Now on to me. Sunday and Monday went OK. I was much more nauseous than Saturday. I even took chemo naps on both days. (I don't remember the last time I took a nap, so if I call them chemo naps it seems to be easier to fall asleep on those terms than just being tired from my children.) I still have been able to eat some food. My toothpaste tastes horrible, so I decided to stop brushing my teeth and really turn into Uncle Fester. Just kidding! Lynda P., a friend of my brother's, (who has gone through this) sent me toothpaste that worked for her. Smells are getting to me if they are cooked in the kitchen, especially cauliflower (but I was still able to eat it). Reminds me of when I was pregnant.

The last day of summer vacation was a beautiful day. Today, Raney and Becca started on a new venture and I started my new venture - daily walking. New beginnings are a wonderful thing and what a great time to start. Fall is

11

coming up and that is a great season. Winter I might need a little bit of a booster (like a vacation to Florida or somewhere sunny in February) to keep the blahs away. I am a SUNNY person. And I am tired. I was not going to get up this early for school. Too bad they don't have homework. Right now they are watching TV because what else do you do on the first day of school when you don't have to leave until 7:40 am?

Well, I best be off to get something done - at least I will shower before school so I can walk into the building looking presentable (but definitely not awake). Even my morning tea is not tasty. That's sad. I need to find another way to make the world a civilized place.

Have a wonderful day and I will chat later!

Posted Sep 4, 2007 4:15pm

Well, I survived the first day of school, though I am not sure about Raney and Becca - we will see at bedtime. I walked with a friend for about an hour and a half. That was great! Not only was the day beautiful (we walked down by the lake and the million dollar homes) but it sure did keep the nausea away.

I went to my part- time bookkeeping job and had lots to keep me busy (don't tell my boss but I was not as speedy as I have been in the past - been out of practice). I didn't get a nap in today but I am sure the three of us will be hitting the sack early; and I am double checking the alarm! Raney set it for 5:30am and then changed it to 6:30am so she wouldn't get in trouble. The last thing I remember saying to her is, we don't have to get up at 5:30am for an 8:00am start time. Can you tell I am still not thrilled with the 5:30am wake up this morning? Well, we have homework and so the school year begins.

I love the messages and they really do help. And the little gifts are fun too!

Thanks so much!!!!

Well, one week down, 15 to go I think. I survived the first week of school. (175 days until summer break!!) I am tired but walking every morning for about 1.5 hours. We (some of the local ladies have been joining me) walk about 4 miles. I feel my best walking but by the afternoon I am tired. The nausea seems to be lessening but it is still there. I am still able to eat. Tonight I made dinner, thanks to my brother-in-law's delivery. The carrots tasted like carrots. That was nice. Dinner was tasty. I am still going to avoid my toothpaste and use this other toothpaste. I am not sure I will be able to go back to my Colgate or morning tea.

Besides walking, I went and saw an acupuncturist. She inserted 12 needles. One she said was to make the tumors shrink - and that one I did feel, even now I can still feel the point. I am hoping it does the job. I would love to shock the doctors and have them wonder, "Where did the cancer go?" Until then I am scheduled for chemo on Friday the 14th (my 40th birthday).

I think the second treatment won't be as easy in the sense that now I know how I feel afterwards. It is getting long already. All the cards, emails, comments on Care Pages, and most definitely prayers and thoughts are keeping me going. I couldn't do this alone and even though I haven't contacted each person individually, everything is so appreciated. I think about all of you all day long. I will never be able to thank you enough for walking this journey with me. In my future life I will find a way to say thanks, but my present life limits me with the amount of energy I am offered daily (which is hard to accept). But I know this is temporary.

Wednesday is the big day for the haircut. Maybe I will buy a new outfit for the occasion! Send suggestions.

Well, Raney just got home from ice-skating and I need to get her to bed. Thanks again for all your kindness.
(And added goodnight, Love Raney)

Good evening. Today was Becca's first gymnastics meet in Racine and I made it. Rob took Becca the hour and 45 min before the meet time and my brother, Jimee, picked Raney and I up and we made it on time!! This was great because I didn't have to rush, like in the past, for my shower and breakfast. Becca had her best meet so far in her life today.

But I am a mean mommy! Poor Raney complained of a sore throat and I still made her go watch her sister. She fell asleep while driving home - not a good sign.

To make a long story short, Raney has strep and Rob tells me I need to call my oncologist. I am not sure why; I am just tired and nauseas, no sore throat, but I made the call. Ten minutes after discussing white blood counts, chemo, and asking me something that sounded very personal - "Are you v...?" (that means being more susceptible to infections for those with naughty minds) which I don't think I am, I now have to take my temperature 4 times a day until my next blood count. That is on Friday. I remember the simple life of strep when it only affected the kids and not me.

I even kissed Raney good-bye today when I went to the store without thinking I might catch something that could send me to the emergency room. I have a long way to go to stay clear of germs when my mom taught us to eat them - now I have to run and hide and I have to hide well so Raney and Becca can't find me.

I guess it is time to say good night and sweet dreams. I have been having strange dreams. I need to write them down because last night was really strange but now I can't remember.

Thanks again for all your support.

14

Just a quickie - Becca is now home with strep so I am taking my temperature 8 times a day. Thank goodness I only have the two children or the thermometer would never be out of my mouth - which Raney and Becca would probably like because then I couldn't tell them to clean their rooms!

I am feeling very much like myself; nausea is just on the outskirts, hovering but not in the playfield. My week will be good, and then next week I will have the reinforcements helping me build back my strength and then hopefully another week like this.

Have a wonderful day and thanks again for all your thought and prayers.

P.S. Wednesday at 6:15 pm my haircutting party begins! Anyone is welcome to join.

The countdown begins for the haircut but I need to share a quick story. I made a regular Doctors' appointment today in case I need a local one. I mentioned that Raney and Becca have strep and that I need to take my temperature 4xdaily - which has been normal each and every time - and you know what he said!!? "We need to give you a strep test in case you are a carrier." The strep virus strikes again. I have no symptoms and still get gagged. I am not sure of the results yet; I was able to leave before the test was done.

I will write again on how the haircutting party went. From what I understand, it involves lots of wine and little hair...

The deed is done! I am wearing a pink Bears hat - compliment of my Packer-fan neighbor. My head is cold so I am very happy to have a hat. I love the way the haircut feels. I told my neighbor from Gurnee, who was at the party, how I loved to feel her boys' hair when they get the summer crew haircut. Now I don't have to hunt crew cut heads down anymore. I just take off my hat.

When everything was gone but my bangs, Lori (the hair cutter) told me to go compose myself. I didn't think I needed composing. I wasn't sobbing or even crying, so I said, "I don't need composing so keep going." I think if I had listened to her and looked I would be having bangs right now. Then I would only be G Jane and I want GI Jane - so off went the bangs!

And as Rob put it (after I asked him what he honestly thought), "It isn't a sexy haircut, but it's not bad." So there you have it. I have a "not bad" haircut.

I am not sure how many days I have to get used to this new 'do before I lose all my hair, but I probably will need more time than I'll get. I won't be crying myself to sleep tonight. It really is an OK haircut. I have pictures so I hope to figure out how to post this weekend. I don't think that I look anything like my brothers, so there is still WOMAN left in me.

Two reasons why I am able to do these things with a smile, strength, and courage are: one, I watched my mom for many years and, two, I have the best support system possible.

Again thanks for everything. I couldn't do it alone.
Hugs and Kisses,

Here is to being bald - I need a glass of wine!!

16

Just another quickie. I am tired. Raney totally fell apart on me tonight. I guess a fuzzy-head mama is not comforting.

Someone said to me today that they were not going to ask me what I am doing tomorrow for my birthday, but I will tell you what my 40th is going to be: I am going to the front lines to do battle. I am getting the reinforcements to help me win!!! (Even though they will knock me out next week.)

Until the next update,
Have a great day!!

I survived the big 40 with great dignity. Even though it was my party - and actually the party lasted all day - I didn't cry.

I did my morning walk and used a pedometer that my cousin sent me; I walked over 10, 000 steps on my 40th with my walking group.

A friend drove me to downtown Chicago and we went out to a birthday lunch. My sister met us on the 21st floor for the chemo appointment. We were then joined by my cousin, Jeff, who rode his motorcycle all the way from Peoria (very far south in Illinois). After chemo, we went to Katy and Jimee's for a pizza party. My dad, Kristin (who brought the pizza), Larry, Sharon, and my QT-pie nephew, Aidan, joined my ever-growing party.

After this party, Rob and I came home to another one thrown by Raney, Becca, and Linda. They decorated the house, staged a surprise entrance (Linda was directed by Raney for about 8 minutes on how to alert Becca and her that I was the one walking through the door - not sure who else she thought was going to be at our house that night!) and they made us chocolate chip cookies.

17

Most of my meals were given to me on '40 year-old' plates so I was not able to forget I turned 40!

Let me tell about one of the many gifts (all were wonderful) because I really think that my husband did great. He got me what I will describe as a very feminine robe: long, black, with flowers. I think when I don't feel so feminine I will wear this and feel womanly.

Girls are home from a wedding I will write more later.

Posted Sep 16, 2007 4:25am

Yes, I am awake. I am having a hard time falling back asleep, so therefore I figured I would finish writing about my big 40. Back to the robe - It is not one I would ever buy myself because I don't dress very "girly" (such a word when you are forty!). I really think it is going to come in handy, especially after surgery when I lose probably what one might consider my most feminine (at least outwardly) parts. I might even have to get manicures during this time of my life, and wear make-up every day, and oh no, high heels?!! Maybe the heels are pushing it because they are not comfortable. The possibilities are endless.

I think I forgot to mention the white blood cell shot didn't hurt this time. The trick is to get it room temperature. I tell you, tricks are a very good thing to learn very quickly in this war. I feel like I am winning when there is little pain.

My white counts were higher this time. I went from a 6.9 count to a 7.1. That is with two cases of strep in my house. I am a fighter - no germs coming into my body. I must not be a carrier either because I didn't get a call; always good to know you are not the one infecting your family.

I am not sure about the tumor from a medical standpoint because the doctor was on vacation so there was no measuring, but if you are willing to take my word I think maybe there was shrinkage. My clue is that my bra is leaving fewer indents on me (I know boys, more information than you want but hey, there you have it, not very lady-like, huh? Maybe when I hit my feminine stage my notes will be ladylike.)

Saturday, two of my sisters hung out with me while Rob and the girls went to a wedding, which I heard was wonderful. I am bummed to be missing things like this. I also missed my future sister-in-law's shower/bachelorette day, but I need to listen to my body and know that I will be back out socially again soon. It is hard to be the one who stays home. I had a quiet Saturday and that was nice.

So to sum it up: I am having a very different 40th birthday than I imagined. I mean, come on, it started on a *Friday*. I could have had something going all weekend long! But it is still a wonderful birthday. I am thinking of Antarctica for my 50th so I can be on top of the world (in a way). I have heard from people that I haven't heard from in a long time and am getting lots of prayers that I know are working. My nausea is still at bay and maybe that is the way it will be all week. A gift I would like from God?? No nausea sure would rank high at this point in my life.

Thank you for all your comments. I have so many that I am not able to respond to all, but I am reading them and at the end of this I am going to print and keep my journal with all the notes that I have received because I never want to forget the love and support I am getting on my journey.

Thanks so much - love, Patty - who jumped into the club and the water was warm. It was painless to turn 40. Good night!

Posted Sep 16, 2007 1:30pm

I am shedding.

Yes - I still plan on posting photos. I just need to figure it out. Now I look like Britney Spears in her really bad hair days, just without the headlines!

I will tell you a secret - I was very sad yesterday. My dad went to get the girls after school so I read *I'd Rather Do Chemo Than Clean Out the Garage:: Choosing Laughter over Tears* (highly recommend the book, it is very funny but you do need a sick sense of humor) when I heard other kids walking home from school. I wanted to be the one to get Raney and Becca. It is hard to realize how little energy I have because of something out of my control.

Today is a much better day. I think that the 4-5 days after chemo and the aftermath is hard, but then the upswing is so great that even though I am not at my same level of energy, I have more!! In fact, today Raney and Becca got out of school early and we went on a bike ride. Afterwards we had a picnic on the rocks by Lake Michigan. I told them that on days that I can do things with them, that's what we should do and we should save play-dates for the days I don't have energy. And what could possibly be more fun than pulling out the little hair that is left on your mom's head under the shade of a tree in the park?

I am thinking that by the time that I am 40 years and one week old, I will officially be gray-free! How many of the new 40ers can say that without the use of hair chemicals???? Be honest.

It is a bit rough around the house for Raney and Becca when I am low on energy. I try to maintain normalcy as much as possible, but when I want to go to bed at 5:00pm they do baulk loudly.

Becca told me that she is not sad that I have breast cancer because I am not going to die. I told her that is my goal, but I don't know when God is going to call me home. She has informed me with quite the determination of a Capricorn (Grandma would be proud) that I am not going to die. There you have it. I will be fine. I am walking this path with lots of support and prayers. She still would like me to have hair. I am not pretty (she tells me

20

this, "I am not trying to hurt your feelings but...") so I am using "I am pretty on the inside." We will see if that message sinks in. I am grateful though - I am going to boast now - God did give me pretty eyes so when I have no eyebrows, no lashes, and no hair, my eyes will stand out even more and that's OK. I like the color of my eyes. See, even chemo patients can be vain!

Well, I need to get the girls ready for CCD and the rest of the evening.

Have a great day.

Thanks for all the thoughts and prayers. I am a stronger person because of all of you! Never underestimate the importance of <u>you</u> in my life. Every comment, every thought, every prayer keeps me going in the right direction. I am truly grateful and lucky to have an army behind me. A war cannot be won by one person alone; but with a whole army behind me, we will WIN!!!!

I am back from a weekend getaway to Lake Geneva. There have been 'Patty sightings' outside Kenosha! The ladies at Lake Geneva tell me I am a beautiful bald woman, no scars and a nice shaped noggin. I knew from my baby pictures that I would look stunning of course! But it does help reinforce those beliefs when no one goes running away from me screaming.

Last week – let's see, what I do remember now - well I must have survived because here I am typing to my support group. (And no, I can't say this enough - without your prayers and thoughts this would be so difficult so thank you again.) You all will pass the test at the pearly gates for all the praying you are doing now. I am sure God is quite pleased.

We will skip last week; my dad was here and helped me out with a lot of running the kids back and forth, doing dishes, laundry – you know, all the fun things that come with having a house and kids. Thanks again, Dad.

This weekend we went out to dinner. The road to the restaurant was hilly; yes, Wisconsin has some hills, and the kids loved it. It was like being on a

21

roller coaster! Therefore Great America is out of the question this season. The thought of any ride is enough to triple my nausea.

Sunday (today) Becca had a meet in gymnastics and did well (no state yet but she was closer). (Mothers are allowed to brag, right???)

I am anticipating a very good week. I am almost done with *I'd Rather Do Chemo Than Clean Out the Garage:: Choosing Laughter over Tears*. Humor is the best medicine - it doesn't taste bad, makes you feel good after you laugh, and is one thing you don't mind sharing with everyone.

There was something that I wanted to tell you but for the life of me I cannot remember - this chemo brain is a real drag because I am sure whatever it was it would have made your day. I am sure it was quite poetic or funny or witty - no random, useless, chatting by me. When I am up from 2-4am this morning, I will remember and will let you know.

I am still walking - and have someone with me everyday - so that is a big help.

I am shipping Raney and Becca off to a friend's house and I am going to listen to a funny CD. Humor baby! It is wonderful.

Until our paths cross take care and
thanks again!!!

Posted Sep 24, 2007 11:58am

I remember what I wanted to share with you. Last week one day was quite humid and I needed to wash my face so I went upstairs and started the water, soaped up my hands and started to wash my face, the top of my head and down my neck. When you don't have hair to stop you and you have never washed like this before, there is no stopping your hands. I made quite the mess in the bathroom and called Raney and Becca up to help me clean. I figured in the nine years that I have had them the water never seems to stay in the tub 100%, so they owed me a bathroom clean up. But of course, "Mommy, you don't need to wash your face!" was the last thing they said.

22

Don't you love it? I clean for years and one clean up from them and I am told no messes.

I went on my walk this morning and my ears were a bit cold down by the lake. I understand elsewhere it is quite hot. Not on my side of Kenosha.

This will be a great week. I am feeling so much better than last week. My chemo appointment might be Thursday because the doctor is not going to be at the office on Friday. I am trying to get both on the same day so I only have to go downtown once this week.

Raney, Becca, and I went out to Applebee's last night - Rob was at the Bears game - and they have taken spaghetti off the children's menu. I never knew my children were so inflexible. "It is because Applebee's has the best pasta, Mama, don't you know anything?" said Raney, who noticed that the place wasn't that busy. She added, "It's because the pasta is off the menu and that's what the people come for." Who knew?? But the waitress, noticing the baldness, went to the kitchen and saved the day. The cooks created the pasta dish. So another point for being bald!!! She was given a great tip because of that. Raney wanted to leave her $20 (more than the total cost of dinner).

I am going to eat some lunch.

Enjoy the sunshine and have a great day.

Please feel free to share any funny jokes, comments, or sayings! A group that laughs together stays together, and I want us together for the long haul -together laughing. It makes the load lighter!!!!

Love to all.

(Not my words until the last sentence, but this is great...)

There once was a woman who woke up one morning,
looked in the mirror,
and noticed she had only three hairs on her head.
Well," she said, "I think I'll braid my hair today."
So she did
and
she
had
a
wonderful
day.
The next day she woke up,
looked in the mirror
and saw that she had only two hairs on her head.
"H-M-M," she said,
"I think I'll part my hair down the middle today."
So she did
and
she
had
a
grand
day.
The next day she woke up,
looked in the mirror and noticed that she had only one hair on her head.
"Well," she said,
"today I'm going to wear my hair in a pony tail."
So she did
and
she
had
a
fun,

fun
day.
The next day she woke up,
looked in the mirror and noticed that there wasn't a single hair on her head.
"YEA!" she exclaimed,
"I don't have to fix my hair today!"
Attitude is everything.
Be kinder than necessary, for everyone you meet is fighting some kind of
battle.
Live simply,
Love generously,
Care deeply,
Speak kindly.......
Leave the rest to God
Life isn't about waiting for the storm to pass...
It's about learning to dance in the rain.

Now my turn -
I love to dance with my friends!
Love to all to the moon and back (or maybe I should say Mars since it is here
at the moment).

Posted Sep 26, 2007 7:54am

I wasn't finished getting bald so yesterday I went and had my (what I had
started to call lovely) hairs sheared off. I look much better all bald. You all
would be very impressed. After my haircut, my stylist (who never had to do
this before) washed my head and the water ran down my head towards my
neck. It felt very strange. Then I got my eyebrows done. (I will probably
lose those this weekend after chemo treatment #3).

The cover of my book, when I write one, will be: I Rock as a Bald Woman!!!!! I
will reach millions of women going through this journey, making them laugh!!!

I was styling after my appointment. I looked good enough to be taken out on
the town.

Yesterday in Kenosha we had quite the downpour and I got caught in it. My Betty Boop bandana got soaked. I went upstairs, took a wash cloth, dried my head, put on my Tweety bandana and I was ready to go. I didn't have to worry about my new style at all. It was nice. The benefits of being bald are endless. They are starting to outweigh the need for hair.

I will have to finish my story later... (I am pulling a Steven King here).

Until then,
Have a great day!

Posted Sep 28, 2007 11:22am

OK - I ran out of time for the last story and notice I left some things out. I could try to blame that on the chemo but my husband says I start a lot of conversations halfway through or I never finish my statements. It's hard to believe that *I*, a woman of a million words, do not finish sentences. Most of you get me and my language (except for maybe my "spa" statement – aka chemo treatment - it sounds more fun saying 'I am off to the spa' than 'I'm being poisoned today').

Ok. If I remember correctly, I left you off at the ability to put myself back together in 1 minute after getting caught in a major downpour. I was talking with my neighbor and sharing the story with her. She told me she can't really remember me with hair. She also said that she had a school meeting and she felt her hair was crazy — she was caught in the storm as well - and was debating what to do with her hair (she is usually very put together). I said I don't have those issues anymore. The only thing about my baldness is that I have a tan line - but I look at that as a benefit because then I know where my face stops!

I spent Thursday night at my sister's. My brother picked me up from the train station, ordered Chinese, and we watched Bionic Woman - which I liked. I haven't watched much TV at night since marriage. (Rob and I have one TV in the house because I don't want more. I really don't want to get into the habit of a lot of TV.)

26

It was fun to hang out with my siblings. After Jimee left, Katy and I started to play with a Shrek hat (my brother-in-law ordered this hat through the mail and sent it to Jimee). Katy and I decided that in order for the Shrek hat (made out of nylon so it is slippery on a bald head) to work, you need hair, but we got some good laughs.

Jimee picked me up for my spa treatment @ 6:45a.m., a bit early - too early in my opinion.

After seeing the doctor I was given great news: My evil friend (as I have so lovingly named my tumor) has shrunk 2.1 cm - better than expected!!! Your prayers are part of that accomplishment, please keep them coming. My evil friend sometimes sends me pain, not too often but enough to let me know it's there. But I am getting even. I am kicking it out of the home it is trying to take over. I don't want this tenant so I am doing what I can to kick it out!!! If we keep up this pace I will shrink my evil friend 8.4 cm. Then only .3 would be left cringing in the corner screaming, "What have you done to the rest of me?"

I need to sign off because I have to go to acupuncture now. I will finish the rest of the story later.

Until then, have a wonderful day

Posted Sep 28, 2007 2:18pm

After my spa treatment, Jimee, my dad, and I went out to lunch. I fell asleep on the way home. My child, Becca, was waiting for me with a 102 fever. I, being the paranoid mother, rushed her to the doctor. Becca told me she had a sore throat, so I thought STREP. No such luck - she has a virus and her fever was 103 this morning. I think that strep would be easier because after 24 hours she'd no longer be contagious and she'd feel better; with the virus - until the fever is gone, which I heard can last up to five days - she can be crabby. Here I thought strep was bad!

Today I walked about 3 miles and went to the acupuncturist. Shrinking my evil friend! Boy I feel some of those needles she says are to shrink the evil friend. I believe that it is working, and this is not chemo alone.

Well, that is all the words of wisdom I have today. As I told my brother, I don't think I am as funny for a few days after chemo. I have chemo brain and I am not that thrilled with chemo brain. I am told I will have it for about 2-3 months after chemo, maybe that's a good thing; I might not remember anything about the surgery or the recovery.

There is always positive in the seemingly negative. Or at least that is what I am striving for. I am the only one who can choose my attitude on this journey; how I decide to react will make this easy or hard. I chose easy - so let's keep praying, smiling and trucking!!

I knew there was something else I wanted to share-
When I was in 4th grade I learned to play the clarinet. I played until high school and then let it go; but I have missed it. The other day I went to a music store in Kenosha and bought a notes booklet to remind me of the notes, and I got an exercise book like the one we played in grammar school. I also bought four reeds. I am going to resurrect my clarinet. *I'd Rather Do Chemo Than Clean Out the Garage* talks about getting back to your passion. I think that this is it. I am hoping to get good enough to maybe find a local group to join. Who knows? The sky's the limit and I am getting ready to test the sky.

OK, I think I am done now. My child calls for me.
Thanks for all your love and support

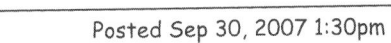

Posted Sep 30, 2007 1:30pm

I finally figured out how to post the pictures from my haircutting party! I will update with the bald pictures pretty soon. I am actually learning to like being bald! As those who know and love me know- which is all of you - I have never been big on the hair regiment in the morning. Now I take a hand towel and wipe my head, grab a bandana or hat, and I am ready for the day. The other bonus: I was told at my last spa treatment that I might not lose all my eyebrows or lashes. This is probably the only time in my life that I liked my bushy eyebrows. I should know by the end of the week if they are going to be staying.

Well I need to get going.
Have a wonderful rest of Sunday!
Thanks again for all your prayers and thoughts - none go unnoticed.

Posted Oct 3, 2007 4:51pm

Hello, Everyone - Raney and Becca are off learning about God at CCD. Raney decided today that she needs to go to Catholic school. I think she wants a new school every year. She is my drama queen. (My mom is laughing at me every day.)

Sunday, Raney and Becca threw a hat, scarf, and bandana party for me with some of my lady friends. Raney was quite nervous about decorating and everything. She even made her own butter for the party. She was very successful so I think that in college she will have no problems throwing some good wing dings! (She is just going to have to get used to her mother being there because I don't have enough of a chemo brain to forget our parties at Marquette. Poor Raney and Becca; I am going to cramp their style and love every minute of it.)

I am not sure how many hats, scarves, or bandanas I received because I am not able to count that high right now (I am still hoping to regain the brain). I didn't get one repeat of anything - even bandana colors. My brother, Budd, gave me a blonde wig and my brother, Ryan, gave me a pink cowgirl hat. Ryan bought himself a cowboy hat awhile ago and I made (just a little bit of) fun of him. Had I known I was going to be bald and he was going to have a chance at pay back, I might not have been so vocal! Then again, who would miss that opportunity?

The day couldn't have been more perfect, and I think that all the ladies did their hair special for me because everyone was radiant! (Or maybe I bring out the best in everyone?!!)

29

My sister, Katy, told me that I was more energized after the party than before. But that is me - a people person. There is nothing better than hanging out with friends, making fun of the Packers, enjoying a glass of wine- -or in my case - water. I have my strength because of everyone and now I am able to reconnect with some lost (but not forgotten) friends. My evil friend has given me the opportunity to re-evaluate what is truly important. Even though I know what is important, somewhere along the path I forgot how to keep it active in my life. I still get impatient with Raney and Becca - especially when I am ready to sleep - but I am remembering what I need to teach them about life - and it is not having the cleanest closet in Kenosha. Sometimes it is hard to remember they are still quite young when they are trying to be so independent, but I am doing my best. I want this path paved with no cracks for when those teenage years are running rampant in my house (wishful thinking I know, but I think I am allowed some delusional thoughts).

I need to send a second update – I've talked too long again.

Posted Oct 3, 2007 4:52pm

The second half of my long winded chatter:

Tuesday I went downtown to get BRAC1 & BRAC2 blood work test done. This will tell me if I am mutated and carry the cancer gene. It is information that will help me decide what to do about surgery and help my girls later in life (and also my brothers and sisters will have a piece of information they can decide what to do with).

I took the train downtown and had lunch with my brother Jimee. Lunch was something I really like, Thai, but this time it didn't have much taste. I think I am going to be very happy when food starts tasting like food again. This is getting to be a drag. I think I am doing OK. I get out everyday - walking or taking the kids here and there. I think Raney and Becca are OK with the baldness now.

According to the oncologist that I met with (I am taking part in a study - all they needed was some blood and I have no problem with trying to help find answers) this is as bad as it will get – I've had some harder days than others but nothing yet that has put me under the table. When I am being carried by friends and family, everything is doable.

I best be off to get the girls and hope they are filled with God's love so there is no fighting tonight. By 6:00pm I am ready to call it a day.

Last night, I snuck upstairs to bed at 7:40pm. I was supposed to go to a card making class but after dinner I was starting to fall asleep at the table. I couldn't tell if I was hot or cold or what was wrong, so I decided I should just go to sleep. Rob sent the girls up around 8:00 with instructions not to wake mommy (of course with them, walking upstairs woke me up). Before Rob hit the last stair Raney was in bed with me and Becca stopped by with children's Tylenol to see if she could take some because she had a headache. (I think she really just needed a kiss goodnight and that was her way of not getting in trouble.) Some habits are hard to break.

I was watching CSI the other day. It was the season premier with a cliff hanger from last year where Sarah was kidnapped. The race to find her in time was basically the whole show. It was quite exciting. As I was watching the police in cars and helicopter swarming the desert - knowing Sarah only had a few precious hours left - I thought, wow, all those people there to help one person. Then I realized that is exactly what I have, all you helping me - just one person! Yes, it is bigger than that because of Raney, Becca and Rob, and bringing good into the universe, but we are a group because of my evil friend. It is very emotional to think of all the love we have to share with one another.

This morning I am full of zip; when you get nine hours of sleep, it helps. I am going for my morning walk which my brother Jimee put on mapyourrun.com. We think it is about a 5 mile walk.

Lol (Lots of love; laugh out loud; living out loud - you decide...)

31

My sister is looking for a superhero name for me. Here's my vote: Chemo Brain! She wears pink from top to bottom. She will mess up dates and 4th grade math, but always with a smile because she can't remember anything so there is nothing to be unhappy about.

I need a groundhog day where I get to redo today. I got up at 6:00am, put on a pair of pink sweats (to be comfortable), a pink hat and a pink bandana (because at 6:00am that seems like a good idea). I woke the kids and had them ready for school 45 minutes early. I then left the house and drove to Waukegan to catch the 9:10am train to be downtown for a 10:30am doctor's appointment. I had gone to the 21st floor to find out where my appointment was because the floor that I went to said there was no appointment for me. The woman told me the appointment is for the 15th - I almost cried.

After I composed myself and left the office I did what a woman does in Chicago with no kids and no husband. Shop!!!! Actually, I only went into two stores. I am really such a non-shopper. As I was walking back to the train station and saw my reflection many times over, I realized I look like a poster woman for Breast Cancer; a little much with the pink from head to toe. Next time I think I will let my children dress me when I get up that early. I did get a free bottle of water because the Chicago Marathon is happening at some point this month. Therefore I need to realize my day wasn't completely lost.

I did a project on the train and started to read a book, so I enjoyed my train ride.

There you have it-
A day with Chemo Brain!! The comics are going to sell millions.
Anyone read the Stephan King pop-up book? I can't remember the title. I think it is for kids. I thought it might be fun to start my kids reading Stephan King at 9 and 7. I think their dreams need a little help.
Have a wonderful weekend--

Lol

Hello, everyone,

Let's see--I think I am still in denial and very slow. The other day I was thinking how for the rest of my life the fear that my evil friend might return in some other shape or form will be with me, in the back of my mind. I am not going to hide from this fear or let it win by not living. But every day will be viewed differently than in my past. I had a shift in my life when my brother Kevin died, so it's not always a bad thing to re-evaluate the importance of living. No more ruts for me!!

This past weekend we just hung around Kenosha and had a quiet weekend. Raney and I rode bikes down to the harbor market and purchased some soaps and fresh veggies. Sunday, the kids played all day. Raney even rearranged her room. I guess when you are nine it is important to be the one who decides where the bed goes. I can't remember that, but I do remember picking out my carpet.

I remember what I wanted to share. I received about 15 bandanas - so now when I get dressed in the morning - if it is not a hat day - I have to coordinate my bandana with my outfit. It is quite funny sometimes because I will catch myself after about 5 minutes realizing I need to get going. Thank God my hairless head doesn't take me any time (except for when I fall back into the habit of leaving the conditioner on for 3-5 minutes, you know, so I am tangle-free!).

I just wanted to say chemo treatment Number 4 is this Friday and then we are halfway through. The next four treatments I switch cocktails so I am back to the unknown, but I think it will be easier for some reason.

I need to get Raney. Have a wonderful evening and I will chat again soon.

Good Afternoon - See I am getting better, I know what time of the day it is! We went out to dinner last night at *Italian Kitchen*. When the girls and I sat

33

down, Rob looked at me and said something about taking off my hat, and then he said never mind. I think he forgot for a moment that I am bald. Maybe he will like this look because I love the convenience.

This restaurant, in Deerfield, is where we are having Jimee and Kristin's wedding shower this Saturday. The menu was not decided yet, so I thought going to dinner would be a great way to get that done. This restaurant was open in 1968 and is family-owned. Awesome food!! In speaking with the mom of the business, she asks me "Is it here or out?" (Meaning catering.) I have spoken to Mary two times and she always says,"OK, we will get it together, no problems." Most people would have freaked, but not me!! I stayed calm and went home full and satisfied with a very delicious meal in my belly (add enough garlic and I can taste!!).

I called Johnny today - he is the son that is taking over the restaurant and is back from vacation just in time to take care of the menu and shower. I would love to share with you what will be served but I am not 100% sure. I told Johnny no shellfish and a veggie dish to take care of a few family members. We are good to go!!

Rob told me last night and this morning that I looked tired. Black circles under the eyes. (I guess staying up to watch the Bears beat the Packers on Sunday wasn't in my best interest since I still haven't caught up on my sleep, but it was a lot of fun!!) He needs a class about how to compliment the wife. I dressed up (for me) last night. I even had on matching earrings, necklace and bracelet. He said I should take a nap today. Now that is probably the first time, even with two kids 20 months apart, that Rob has ever said for me to nap. I almost went into shock. The problem with napping is I am afraid it will keep me up at night. I probably fell asleep within five minutes last night and then I didn't wake up and stay up in the middle of the night like I had before.

The other night Raney got all mad at me because I won't give a nine-year-old a cell phone. I can't imagine the conversation when I say no to the computer and telephone in her room. I am so old fashioned. "Everyone has a cell phone, MOM!!!" There are three people in her class with phones - once I got the truth out of her. I guess letting her move her room around and giving her a little decision power has gone straight to her head.

34

I have been waking up without my hat on so I don't know if I am getting hot while I am sleeping or if the hat is slipping, but I told the acupuncturist that I am walking up bald because there is no hat on, not because there is no hair.

Too long of a message again so another to be continued...

Posted Oct 11, 2007 1:36pm

And now back to the rest of the story

Tomorrow I am half-way through CHEMO!!! I am getting tired of the tiredness and nausea - I won't miss that at all. I won't lie; it gets to be a real drag. I have harder days than some. I do try to keep my chin up and stay positive but sometimes my evil friend gets the best of me. Luckily I think it is just a small amount (unless I am in denial and my family would tell you a different story!).

I went to acupuncture today because of the shower on Saturday. She put a needle in my 3rd eye today. It is in the middle of your forehead, the charka point that has to do with emotions. We will see. If I start bawling at chemo tomorrow because I am dreading what is to come then I will know I am in touch with my emotions.

I think that is what is new with me. I had a pretty quiet week last week. I hope all is well with everyone and you are enjoying the fall weather. I am watching the trees on my walk and it is fun to see the quick changes on some trees and then the others that just don't seem to want to believe winter is on its way.

Thanks again for all your thoughts and prayers. I am excited to see how much more my evil friend has shrunk. I will keep you posted.
Until the next posting have some fun!!
Love to all

Once again I am up at the ungodly hour. Raney and Becca are having a sleepover with Aunt Eileen downstairs, so no one has been able to bother me with bathroom breaks or nightmares or "I heard a sound..." I can only blame myself for not being able to turn my brain off.

Friday my last of the tough chemo went well. My friend, Lori, drove me downtown Chicago, my sister, Eileen, met us on the 21st floor, Rob took a half a day off and my nieces, Angi and Andrea, ventured on the EL to meet us. During this time we were putting together cards for the shower that was happening the next day. Lori took a couple sets of cards home with her and we did the rest during plug-in time. Afterwards we went to see Angi and Andrea's apartment in the city. Two bathrooms, three bedrooms; very cool apartment. We went out to dinner at a Thai restaurant. It was a nice evening catching up. I fell asleep on the way home and my children were waiting for me to say goodnight. A friend stopped by with the envelopes for the cards and I sent another set of cards home with her - all together we made 200 cards - Raney, Becca, my dad, my sisters, Lori and Ann.

I got busted by Rob so I am going to try and go back to sleep. I will finish tomorrow.

I hope you like the pictures from the hat party. It was a great time.
Talk to you in a few hours.

I didn't get back as soon as I thought but here I am. The shower went off without a hitch so that is a good thing.

Sunday was just a lazy day but I did get a birthday gift 5 days early for Becca's friend. I am telling you, this is really the way to live. No rushing at the last minute. Just don't tell Ann W. that is my new way of life as she was here Saturday wrapping the shower gift minutes before we were to leave.

36

Today was an appointment - on the right day - and I didn't wear one stitch of pink. After doing laundry I noticed that the pink sweats that I wore on my last outing to downtown by myself didn't just say "Las Vegas" like I thought - but across the butt stated, "That's Hot-Las Vegas." How embarrassing!!

No free water today - they ran out during the Chicago Marathon.

Raney cried last night because she wanted to go with me to the doctor's instead of school. There was no good-bye from her today. I can't imagine what she is going to be like as a preteen and teenager. I think going through chemo is going to be a lot easier than dealing with teenagers.

I can't believe I forgot this bit of news!!
I'm shrinking. Last time I missed some numbers which worked out because they were 6x6.6 - not to be all about the devil, but those are not my favorite numbers. This week I am 4.5x5.5. I almost back to normal.

To my lady friends: It is time to feel yourself up! Breast Awareness Month. Let's make sure that we are taking care of ourselves so that we can live to ripe old ages and talk about how I am a perky old lady!!! No sagging here!!! My hair might come back with no grays, so no more highlighting. Think of all the money I could save.

I need to get the evening going so I will chat later
Have a wonderful evening.
Thanks again for all your support.

Posted Oct 17, 2007 12:07pm

This morning my nausea and tiredness is in its prime. Thank God this should be the last of feeling this way. Rob tells me this morning that I seem crabby and short with my preteen (yes at nine she is preteen and loving every moment of arguing and yelling at me). I can't remember what else he said but then sarcasm slipped out. I said, "I guess I am tired of being nauseas, tired, bald and sick." I think that my family is in denial. What part of this journey do I like?? I know that at the end things will be better and that this is not something that is going to beat me, but it does win some of the moments. I am trying to do all the right things but sometimes it is a heavy load.

I tell you when I was in Heaven signing up for my life sessions I guess I forgot to read the fine print on this one. Serves me right, I was probably gabbing with the soul next to me. I wonder what they ended up getting in this lifetime.

I heard on the radio today that acupuncture helps with pain control after surgery and nausea with chemo - a study by Duke University. If I am this nauseated for a week after chemo with acupuncture, I wonder what it would be like with no acupuncture.

What I am really getting tired of is food not tasting good, and nothing makes the stomach feel ok.

I am grouchy today and it's a beautiful day. I think I need to get off my bandwagon and go to my Zen room and refocus on the positives. I have so many people behind me and that is what is really important. I am not alone and, as long as they keep the laws the same, my husband is safe as well - telling me I am crabby. He needs a class on what to say and what not to say to his bald wife.

OK, enough - I promise I will be good.
Off to Zen and peace

Have a great day.

Posted Oct 19, 2007 7:29am

So another evening of getting up to go to the bathroom about 4 times and trying to regulate my body temperature, which can be difficult when Becca radiates heat to the gazillionth degree. Rob thinks I am not getting enough sleep, but aren't bags under the eyes a mother trait?

I went to acupuncture yesterday and she put in gentle needles everywhere, except for the shrinking points. She said I looked weak. I am not sure about that, but I was tired. She put one in the third eye again and I threw the needle. I guess my third eye doesn't want to be poked, but then again what eye wants to be poked?

We are going to take the kids to Gilda's Club this Saturday. They are having a Halloween party. They have a 10 week program that I would like to get Raney and Becca involved in as much as possible. I need them to be around other kids who are going through the same thing so maybe they can figure out what they need to express.

I have to get the girls ready and I am going to watch Raney's patriotic play at school this morning.

Have a wonderful day and I will chat again soon.

Posted Oct 22, 2007 1:32pm

I am thinking of taking the medicine that is supposed to help me sleep because I am getting really tired. I would have been writing last night if Rob wasn't upstairs wanting to know my every move. Every time I went to the bathroom, "Are you OK? Is there something wrong?" He would not have been happy if I told him I was going downstairs to write my deepest thoughts. That is, if I can find them, I will write them.

Saturday didn't go as planned. We never made it to Gilda's Club. I am not sure that is going to be an option; it is a bit far (1.5 hrs) from Kenosha with no traffic. I am going to a place called the Wellness Center in Northbrook on Thursday, so hopefully there is something there that will help me learn to talk to my girls in a way that they get – or someone else who can.

Sunday, Becca had a meet by the airport in Milwaukee. We went up early and had breakfast with Rob's cousins and then hung outside until it was time to go. It was so nice to relax outside. The weather was great - and so was the company. Becca, by the way, was only .4 points away from qualifying for state. Hopefully next time she will get the 33 points that she needs.

39

Last week was probably the hardest week for me so far with the energy level and that nausea, but I was still able to eat. I have been very lucky in this process. My port causes me no problems; I have no mouth sores; I am able to eat - food doesn't taste good but at least I am eating; I have walking buddies to keep me motivated; people are providing the family with food; friends are donating to Merry Maids. And everyone keeps praying for me. What more can I ask for? So thank you! Because of you, I am able to feel lucky.

I just want to stay focused on the good and let the bad fall to the wayside. I was told by a woman who went through chemo that treatment number 4 was a very difficult one but that it does get better. I am nervous about the next four - even though I am told the nausea won't be as bad, the tiredness is really supposed to be pronounced. I am not sure I will be able to manage being more tired than I already am. I will have to wait and see about that. Thank God that it only takes me two seconds to dry my head! And ladies, I don't think that I have been bragging enough about saving time also by not needing to shave anywhere on the body, and I get to sleep in to the last possible minute with my new body.

Becca was kind enough to tell me today that I still have a belly. I think I need to kick her out of my room when I am getting dressed. Maybe when they take the ladies I will ask for a few pounds from the belly to go along with them??

What we have going on: 27 days before my brother's wedding. That will be fun. Raney is going to be in a play and Becca has two more meets.

Of course, I get to answer the door at Halloween!!! I might be Uncle Fester or I might just answer the door bald. I am thinking that might scare the little ones - hehehhehehe. I am not sure what the teenagers will think because I don't think anyone knows what teenagers think.

I better boogie and get a few more things done. If only I could remember what it is that I want to get done?

Thanks again for everything and I will chat again soon.

Today I woke up about 2.5 pounds lighter - I had a colonoscopy so I got a nap on the way to Chicago, nap during the procedure, and a nap on the way home.

The stuff they make you drink!! I don't even know what to say about that *!?$*.

Raney, Becca and I watched *Cars* upstairs (thanks to my brother Ryan for lending me his DVD) so I wasn't very far away from my new best friend (we have no bathroom on the main floor). I hadn't seen *Cars* before. I thought it was very cute. Tipping the tractors; how funny was that?

Anyway, I was given a clean bill of health and now I am having fun filling up what was cleaned out!!!!!!!!!!!!!!!!!!!

I didn't get hungry until after the procedure, and it took us 2.5 hours to get home. I was not a pleasant passenger, except during nap time.

I am going to eat more so I will chat later.
Chow
from Cleaned out Patty

Good Morning,
I don't have much time because Rob is working out of the house. Friday begins 'The new Chemo'. They had to give me Benadryl to offset the effects of the chemo, which I did not like at all. It was a strange feeling and I am not sure how to describe it. I also fell asleep (I think for about 45 min) but I guess that wasn't so bad since it took 3.5 hrs once I got plugged in for the poison to run through my veins. There is supposed to be little-to-no nausea so that is a very happy thought. I was really getting tired of that feeling. I might have aches and pains in my bones for a few days afterwards. I had the nurse measure me on Friday and her measurements were a little larger than

the doctor's last measurements. Nothing that alarmed them, but I prefer to think of my evil friend as getting smaller and smaller.

I am going to eat breakfast so I will chat later
3 treatments to go!!!

Posted Oct 29, 2007 1:23pm

I have a few more minutes to update on some of last week. What I can remember, you will read about; what I don't remember, you will read about when some night when I can't sleep and my brain seems to work quite well because it won't turn off.

There was at least one day (I really think only one day) where going up and down the stairs was very tiring. My heart was pounding and I was breathing heavy. I would have thought that I hadn't moved my body in years with how difficult it was. I mentioned it to Rob but that was about it (and those who don't know, we don't have a bathroom on the main floor so I had to go up and down several times) but I didn't call the doctor. I didn't think about it. I still did my walks and that was fine so who knew my red blood counts were dropping.

I think that I should have been given a course before chemo to teach me about all these things that change and are now important to my new life (i.e. taking my temperature with strep, huffing and puffing, etc.) These are things I now need to be aware of and may mean a call to the doctor.

Friday at chemo the nurse asked me about my week - I was busted. I told her that I was short of breath and the whole story. She was surprised that I could still do my walks, but last week I didn't walk Tuesday, Thursday, or Friday (Raney and Becca had the last two days off) maybe that is why I was able to walk. She said that I had to get a shot - in the stomach!! (But it was less painful then in the arm, I was very surprised.) I was bummed that I had to get a shot because it was going to be the first chemo without a shot to boost red or white cells. Maybe next time.

I told you about the chemo and needing naps. My sister, Linda, took the girls shopping around Chicago and my sister, Eileen, hung out with me in my room.

42

Raney and Becca (with Linda) bought me PJs and slippers. It was so funny to see the three of them walk into the room with bags from their shopping spree - very Chicago. Afterwards we went to my brother Larry's for dinner and visited with Aidan who had turned 2 the day before. He is so funny. When we were leaving, we were downstairs in the garage and Aidan was showing us his gymnastics. I put his hood on to protect his head so Becca took my bandana to protect her head. I wish I had a camera to catch the look Aidan gave me when he saw me bald - it was hysterical.

Saturday, we went up to Madison because Becca had a meet there on Sunday. She qualified for state and placed third so she also got a trophy. She was thrilled. When we got home we went trick-or-treating Sunday. That was our weekend.

I am a bit tired this morning. I slept really well last night and in Madison. I don't feel nauseas but my bones hurt more than before, so hopefully that is only a day or two. That is a side effect of this new chemo. And my evil friend shoots pain at me every once in awhile to let me know he is still there. He makes me nervous. I want him gone!!!! I talk to the surgeon in December. I need to get a couple of things done before Raney and Becca get out of school.

Hope all is well with everyone and Happy Halloween!!

P.S. First time that I can remember that I didn't eat candy on Halloween. Candy doesn't taste good at this time. I am not sure if that makes me happy or sad. I used to eat way more then I needed, so it is probably better that I don't like it now.

Posted Oct 30, 2007 5:24pm

OK, today I went for my walk as usual. What a beautiful day in Kenosha. The leaves are brilliant and it was pretty warm down by the lake. I am hoping for a warm November so we can still walk by the lake. After the walk, I was watching this DVD with my dad. I couldn't keep my eyes open so I went and took a 2.5 hour nap. I guess this round of chemo is going to keep my energy down more than the last four treatments. I won't like that but I will listen to what I need to do to grow old. I want to be the sexiest grandma in town since there will be no sagging for me!!!!

This chemo also seems to make my skin more fragile. I was putting together a Halloween treat for Becca's class: 3 dum-dum suckers with orange and black ribbon tied around the sticks. This gave me a blister on my middle finger. And I have quite a number of blisters on my feet from walking. I did not turn forty very gracefully, that's for sure. I am falling apart. But when I am 50 and everything is put back together - like the bionic woman - I will strut my stuff!!! (And pray that nothing falls off.)

But that's it for today.

I hope all is well and everyone gets treats and no tricks for Halloween!! I get to wear my cross and bones scarf tomorrow!!! The kids love it. They think that I look cool--better than being called an old lady like my Becca likes to call me.

Have a great day.

Posted Nov 3, 2007 7:38am

Good Morning
I am as bad as the kids. Saturday is a day to sleep in - especially with the darkness in the morning - and here I am up and ready to greet the day even with Raney and Becca spending the night next door.

I asked a child once why they were easier to get up on the weekend than during the week for school. She answered, because the weekend was free to play and she didn't want to miss a minute of it. The wisdom of children is always amazing to me.

I last spoke on Oct 30th. Let me look at my day timer to see what I have been doing this week since I can't remember. I missed a chiropractic appointment and I forgot to turn Boston coupon books into school. I am batting a 1000. Maybe I should get on the Cubs team and help them out?? I had a quiet week but last night was an outing.

I went out to dinner with a couple of friends. We went to this event called The Power of the Purses. It funds a Woman's Fund in Kenosha that helps out many different areas for women in need. I stayed up past my bedtime of 8:30p.m. I skipped the dessert table (some of my friends would be shocked to actually see that since there was a time in my life that I would eat snickers and drink Pepsi on the way to classes at MU - yuck!!)

At this event they had entertainment. One was Kerri Sherwood, a musician, and the other woman was Karen, Debbie, or Maggie for all I can remember (I have a sheet for Kerri's name). She is an author and a breast cancer survivor. I kept looking at her hair. It was beautiful. I guess I am done being bald. (I am actually ready for this journey to be over, but I still have a ways to go.) She got up and talked a little about her journey. She was saying how when she couldn't see the light at the end of the tunnel, it was her people that always could see the light for her. That is so important.

I have complained to my brother, telling him I am falling apart and that turning 40 wasn't what my friends had emailed and told me: 'the water's fine jump right in', 'turning 40 is great, no problem'. But it still is only for the moment - because we did laugh about falling apart. I will be the bionic woman in the family and if my new ladies (breasts for those that need the actual word) can help in any way to stop a thief or break open a door, I will be there dressed in pink from head to toe.

The two women shared their stories, and then there was music. I told one friend that they better stop with the stories or I was going to start crying. My friend put her hand on me to console me when the lady started talking about when she was told she had breast cancer. I looked over at my other friend and she was sobbing. So what does sensitive Patty do? I started to laugh. Here I am being consoled - not crying - and my other friend is crying and not being consoled. It struck me as funny. I am not sure why. Blame that one on chemo brain as well. Perhaps my third eye needs to be stuck again. Put my emotions back in order.

I also think that I am not going to be able to keep my eyebrows. They are really thinning out. And I keep losing lashes. I may still have a few of those left at the end. It is a race to see what I get to keep before the end of chemo.

My evil friend still shoots pain every once in awhile to let me know he is still there. But he is being served notice and nothing is keeping him here past January. I don't have a date yet. I talk to the surgeon in December.

We have been having great weather in Kenosha. When I begin taking the kids to school there is a tree that looks like it is plugged in when the sun hits it - it is so bright and beautiful. I am going to miss that when the leaves fall off. There are a few trees that I keep watching on my walk. We are still walking by the lake but sometimes when that wind picks up it is cold!!!!

My brother gets married this month and Raney is counting down. She is so excited. She also wants to sit in the front seat of the car and get a cell phone. She is growing up way too fast.

Have a wonderful weekend and I will chat again soon!!

Posted Nov 4, 2007 12:10pm

Yesterday, I went to a restaurant that, as a child, we used to go to all the time for my baby brother's birthday (Ryan!!) and I wore my pink cowboy hat just for the occasion. Ryan was the giver of the cowboy hat. Some lady said that it looked good on me.

What I really want to share with you is that when I was telling the story that I had blogged yesterday to my sister and my dad that I remembered the lady's name - the breast cancer survivor - her name is Heidi!! So if you have patience I will remember things - it just might take me 24 hours or so. I should probably move out west where the pace is a lot slower than the Chicago-land area and then chemo brain wouldn't be as noticeable.

Last night I went to bed about 8-ish. I was very tired from the night before. I asked Rob to send the girls up around 8:30pm - trying to keep a school night schedule even on weekends - then I remembered the time change. I still went to bed but had Rob keep the girls up a little later so there was no

46

6am wake-up from Raney. I had told Becca that she couldn't sleep with me. I thought that I had sent that message to Raney but I felt poking in the arm—"Mama, did I wake you?" When I asked her why she didn't sleep in her own bed like she was suppose to, she said that I only told Becca and that is why she didn't ask me, so I couldn't say no. I tell you someone should write a book to give to parents that will be entering the chemo brain everything that needs to be said to your children so that we are not outsmarted daily.

With our extra hour today we went bowling with about half of Kenosha. We got the last lane available. I did not bowl but cheered on Rob, Raney, and Becca. I produced quite the bowlers.

We are going to enjoy this beautiful day in Kenosha. I hope you all had a great weekend and we will be chatting later.

Love to all

Hi
Someone sent me this email and I thought it was an excellent message - because all of you are getting into Heaven with the way you are helping me out and the universe has become a better place because of it. The real beauty about love and support is that there is no limit to what we can offer the world.

A holy man was having a conversation with the Lord one day and said, "Lord, I would like to know what Heaven and Hell are like."
The Lord led the holy man to two doors.
He opened one of the doors and the holy man looked in. In the middle of the room was a large round table. In the middle of the table was a large pot of stew, which smelled delicious and made the holy man's mouth water.
The people sitting around the table were thin and sickly. They appeared to be famished. They were holding spoons with very long handles that were strapped to their arms and each found it possible to reach into the pot of stew and take a spoonful. But because the handle was longer than their arms, they could not get the spoons back into their mouths.

The holy man shuddered at the sight of their misery and suffering.
The Lord said, "You have seen Hell."They went to the next room and opened
the door. It was exactly the same as the first one. There was the large
round table with the large pot of stew which made the holy man's mouth
water. The people were equipped with the same long-handled spoons, but
here the people were well nourished and plump, laughing and talking. The holy
man said, "I don't understand."
It is simple," said the Lord. "It requires but one skill. You see they have
learned to feed each other, while the greedy think only of themselves."

And all of you are thinking of others as well as yourselves. Thank you so
much for helping me walk this journey because there are days when I am not
a happy camper. I do complain and grouse about being bald, being tired, etc,
etc, etc.

Raney is in a play and she needs to curl her hair. I went and got sponge
rollers and put her hair in them last night - a long story short, she was crying
about her hair this morning and she said I ruined her hair and she wasn't
going to school (the drama of a 4th grader). I got upset and said "At least
you have hair."

One morning Rob was complaining about his thinning hair and that he is going
bald and I said I already was. He said, but yours will come back, and I said
but I am a woman and I shouldn't ever be bald.

I am missing my hair so I don't have any patience for bad hair days in my
family anymore - I'm such a baby! But since I look like an OLD baby I might
as well act like one when people talk about their hair.

I went to my acupuncture appointment on Tuesday. The point to shrink my
evil friend didn't hurt as much this time. I told her that maybe he has
packed his bags and got out of my body. I will find out on Friday. That would
shock the doctors and everyone else - how fun that would be? She did put
some needles in for stress and those hurt more than the other times. I
guess I am a little under stress these days.
My children have a half of day of school so I need to get them lunch - have a
wonderful day and weekend.

Chemo treatment #5 this Friday. I made an appointment with the surgeon December 18th. I will know more about the surgery at that time. Oh, and after the big wedding I will find out if I am to be mutated - I will keep you posted.

Until the next time...

OK, yesterday was a bump-in-the-road day. My friend and I left the Kenosha area around 9:30ish. I thought it would be nice to eat lunch before the spa treatment began - because it is a long one - but Chicago traffic changed all that. We ordered sandwiches and ate in the 21st lobby - the cancer floor. Now the view from the 21st floor is spectacular so it's not the worst place to eat, but not on my top ten places.

I went and had my port put together and the blood is drawn through the port at this time. Last time my red blood counts were low and I was suspicious because I was still a little short of breath and very tired Thursday night but I thought no big deal - the doctor will just do what they did last time. WRONG!!!!! My white blood count: 1.9. My red blood count: 3.1 (and for the medical people who read my blog: Hi, Hi Dr. Lee) my neut # .2. For us non-medical people what this means is not good, no chemo for me. My white counts were too low. Instead I got two shots yesterday (and they were not Jaeger), one for the white blood cells and one for the red blood cells. I guess I should be happy that God didn't give us a rainbow of colors in our blood or I would have gotten 7 shots (if my brain is working, there are 7 colors in the rainbow?). I was lucky enough to have 2 more shots ordered for the rest of the weekend. After the next three chemo treatments, I will have a shot to boost my white blood counts. Instead of having 2 chemos left I am still sitting at three. (With the way my brain has been working, I hope that I remember that I didn't get one and that I show up for my third.)

I was disappointed because I want to keep moving forward and I don't feel like I did that yesterday. Now I go 11/19, 12/7 and 12/21(the last day of school before Christmas break.) The doctor was very calm about this so I take it that this is not an unusual happening. I still feel very blessed with all the love and support that I am getting. I just wish that I didn't have any bumps in the road. It was smooth sailing until yesterday. We will continue to move forward. My evil friend has shrunk some more. I think the doctor said 4x5. I also had the surgeon appointment scheduled for 12/18 but I need to change that because I don't think he wants to see me until I am done with chemo. I might have a day during Christmas break in the decorated city with Raney and Becca, with a doctor appointment thrown into the mix. See positives everywhere. I just have to remember to know they are there.

Becca and the family (with Aunt Linda) are at a meet today. I asked a friend (who also is a dr.) if I would be running a risk going today and she said yes - so I am at home self-nurturing but bumming because this is the first meet I have missed. But I would rather be at home than in the hospital if I were to catch something and not be able to fight it off. I know that my body is not healing as quickly as in the past because the blister that I got at Halloween is still bothering me and not completely healed.

Besides all of that, I laughed a lot yesterday! My brother Jimee and my sister-in-law Kristen got me a Maxine book - and they are hilarious. I was crying I was laughing so hard. I went out to dinner with my sister Eileen and my friend Carrie (my driver for the day). It was a good day even with the bump in the road.

I am going to rest and listen to the silence of the house--

Have a wonderful weekend and enjoy raking if you are lucky enough to have trees in your yard like us. We have at least 3,546,781 leaves that need to be raked, and more on the trees to still fall. Truly a never-ending raking project.

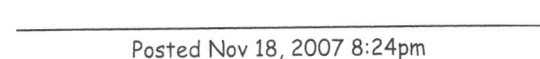

Posted Nov 18, 2007 8:24pm

It has been a long week getting ready for Raney's play opening and the big wedding. I can't remember anything I was going to say about last week so I am going to make the assumption that everything was fine. I am sure that I was more tired than usual, but not so bad that I couldn't get whatever needed to get done, done.

We will talk about Raney's play first. Her opening act was Wednesday and we had a good time. She was a townsperson and the play was about 1.5 hrs. We got home about 9:30ish.

Now on to the wedding weekend!! Friday I went and got a manicure. I figured I may as well look as girly as possible since I wouldn't be able to do a thing with my hair! (Or lack thereof!) Katy and I went around town and finished up the last few errands before the big rehearsal. We went to the hotel and the weekend began (and we are still in the weekend with Becca at a meet right now and Raney doing homework). The rehearsal dinner was at a place called The Barn. I didn't wear the wig there and when I would get hot flashes I would strip off my hat. I am thinking that hot flashes should only happen once in a woman's life. I was one of the last ones from my college group to turn 40, but now I am experiencing something that we new 40-year-olds shouldn't even be talking about yet. Not the new frontier that I was looking to be the one to venture to first, but it is what it is.

Back to The Barn. It was very spacious and fun. They ordered double-decker pizza, and no party can go wrong with good pizza. Even though the place was rocking until midnight, Rob and I left with the kids around 9ish. I am not allowed to write what they did to the cream puffs because young people read the blog but I understand that there were no puffs left by the time the party ended. I was asleep around 10ish. I woke up at 6am and realized I had a morning that I could have slept in! The kids stayed in Aunt Katy and Aunt Eileen's room, so I went back to sleep until 8am.

Then the madness began: breakfast, lunch, hair appointments (Raney and Becca, not me), dressing, make-up, looking for bobby pins, the list goes on and on and on. We made it to the church on time. It was a great ceremony. The ceremony was in the church where I grew up going to mass. We had some time between the mass and reception so we went back to the hotel. During this time, Raney and Becca were with the wedding party, so though my kids were there, I saw very little of them during the day.

As you can gather from the little that I wrote, it was a long weekend and Becca just got home from her meet so we are going to bed. School tomorrow, #6 chemo, we hope, and then we are getting ready to go to Northern WI for the rest of the week. It might be awhile for the rest of the story. But I am doing OK. I have a small cold and I lost my voice but I had a great time at the wedding and I will be relaxing over Thanksgiving by a fireplace.

So until I can write again, have a great day and Happy Thanksgiving!!!!! I have a lot to be thankful for this year because of all the love and support that I have been getting since I started my new journey. I will toast to all of you with my H2O martini on the rocks.

LOL and LOL

Posted Nov 20, 2007 7:10am

Today we are getting in the car to go find snow and cold.

I did want to let you know that chemo was successful yesterday and the Benadryl didn't bother me at all. I had a different nurse and she didn't know to cut the Benadryl in half. When she told me this would delay the starting time I said forget it. We didn't get into a room, I don't think, until 3:40ish and I was ready to rumble!! It took about four hours from start to finish. When I went to the bathroom (I had just woken up from a nap and was a bit groggy) I felt like I was in a mall after hours. I asked my sister if anyone was left to unplug me. It is kind of creepy, hospital silence. I still had 4 people with me so I was not alone - thank God!!

Everyone: enjoy turkey if that's what you eat and have a wonderful holiday. And Jimee and Kristin, if you read this before you leave, bring home sun and sand for us!!!

Talk to you soon.

Posted Nov 29, 2007 8:54am

Rob is out of the house today and I have a few minutes before I walk in 5 degree weather. I am not sure how you people exercise so much - if that is you. I sometimes find it hard to go out and walk. I am so lucky that I have people who join me - I am not sure how much walking I would be doing on my own.

One thing before I go back to the wedding story - which now seems so long ago. A friend of the family sent me a newspaper clipping about a contest that Serta is having. I could win a $10,000 make-over for my bedroom (a king size bed!!!!). I am not sure what they could do in my room that would cost $10,000 because it isn't that big, but perhaps they could find a way to expand my closet!!! I would have to write "how having breast cancer has changed my life" but, here is the kicker, in 150 words!! I am not sure that I can sum up my story in 150 words, being the chatty person I am. I have been thinking about it all month so I am going to give it a shot - I can't win if I don't enter. Once I write my condensed story, I will share it with you.

Back to the wedding: The ceremony was very nice and in the church that I grew up going to. The reception hall had the biggest dance floor that I remember seeing - and I love to dance wild and crazy - but not at this reception. The food was great - my taste buds are mostly back but sometimes I have no interest in food; and my insane brother, Jimee, is back to being normal. He gave up chocolate one year for New Year's and never went back - for 19 YEARS!!! I couldn't give up chocolate for 2 days in my past life. But Jimee ate a piece of Franco Mints at his head table (I might have told you this already. I don't remember.) Now we can go back to having chocolate cake at birthdays!!!!

Jimee asked me to dance, or said he would get a chair and dance with me that way. I was not sure that I would have the energy so I told him it needed to be a slower dance. So off to the dance floor we went. I think that being around people gives me a lot of energy because after that dance I think I went out on the dance floor about 3 more times. I just stood there and moved my arms but it was fun. The other thing about not being on the dance floor is there is a lot more socializing - all the way to Cinderella's time! My children thought they were going to ride back with the wedding party so they didn't want to leave, and I was doing OK so we stayed and stayed and stayed. I didn't want to leave even when we did but I thought it probably was in my best interest to go before the good-byes started to really happen. (If you have ever been around for a Dunn good-bye you know what I mean...they take forever!)

By talking so much and staying out past my bedtime, the next day I didn't have much of a voice left. But we survived. Monday morning was a nightmare trying to get the kids ready for school, but we are completely recovered now - a week in Northern WI helped us out.

Thanksgiving week was very nice. We got up there Tuesday afternoon and stayed until Saturday morning. We went to bed when we were tired - sometimes I went to bed before the kids - and woke up on our own. No structure and no stairs; two great ways for me to get rested. The kids went swimming at the Beacons Resort. I fell asleep poolside. I must have been tired because indoor pools are not the quietest things!

Thanksgiving Day I think I was in my PJs until noon. I watched the Macy's parade start to finish, and then there was a dog show afterwards. The cable up there doesn't have Fox, so Rob had to go to a bar to watch the Packer's game. I don't think I saw any football on Turkey day nor did I cook or clean dishes. I was very pampered!!!! And the dinner was awesome! I will be back next year!!

Well, I better go walk and get that done. It is still 5 degrees!!
Have a great day
LOL

One more quickie--
I went to a breast cancer survivor network yesterday. I was the youngest one there by at least 10 years, so I am going to see if I can find a younger group. I would like to talk to people in the same stage of life if possible (young children at home).

But three of the women are going to Northwestern and all had Dr. Bethke as their surgeon. I am not the only one who drives - or is driven - a very long way for treatment.

They also talked about radiation and helped with some of my fears that I

54

have gotten from reading stories. As for surgery, no one did reconstruction because of their age, so I couldn't gather information about that but I still have some time.

OK, shift gears, I knew that I had a story to tell-

Tuesday morning I had a race with the girls to get ready for school. Raney asked if hair was included and I said yes. After about ten seconds she said, 'that's not fair, you don't have hair!' And I said, 'yep, that's right, and hair is still in the race.'

This weekend we are going to WI Dells for Becca's state meet. We are staying at a water park so I am hoping to go down 8 slides. I guess the place has 8 large water slides. I might only make one with the stairs but we will see. I will let you know how it turns out.

I need to get going before I chicken out because it is still 5 degrees. How I miss the summer sun!!!

Chat with you later
Enjoy your day

Posted Nov 30, 2007 7:54am

OK, another quickie: Rob had the weather bug set to Boulder Junction, WI -- which is 6 hours north - so Kenosha was not 5 degrees (but you could have fooled me) yesterday. I am so gullible.

I (with the help of family) finished my essay for my new bedroom. So send light to the letter today!!!! Next month I will be sleeping in a King size bed!!!!!

Have a great day

I am quite gabby this week! I just finish submitting the winning essay on the Serta website. The contest was with Susan G Kolmen, so it is a "cure" contest. I sent off my version to some of the family. I waited so long that I didn't have time to let everyone look at the essay. I tell you, it is not easy to write something so short when there are so many people that influence how I am able to walk this journey. I feel that there is so much missing in my essay, so what I think I was able to capture was my attitude that I am not going to let cancer keep me from living a life. I am forced to change some of *how* I live but that probably will end up being a good thing; putting the really important things first and letting us wear dirty jeans once in awhile (just kidding I will keep the family clean - at least in public).

But here is the essay and remember, if given the option, it would have been longer to thank all of you again for the thoughts, prayers, meals, cards, car rides, and so much more. THANK YOU!!!!!!

I embrace my pain and baldness...because I am alive.
"You have breast cancer-stage 3." The weight of those words...my choice - let cancer destroy me or beat the cancer. I chose to beat the cancer. And with the help of God, family and friends, I will!!
During chemo, I keep eating though nothing tastes good. Though exhausted, I walk with my friends daily. In pain from head to toe, I watch my children compete in gymnastics and perform in school plays. I am learning life's truly important moments. I am using cancer as my teacher.
I would love a new bedroom design to go with my new body design. Also, more importantly, I would use my new Serta mattress to help me get a complete night's rest.
When I sleep, I heal better.

I find out around Jan. 15th when they are coming to the house to give me a new bedroom!!! Wouldn't that just be so much fun??!!!

Well I need to get the rug rats.
I hope all is well with you and your families

I posted some pictures from the wedding and Thanksgiving. I didn't take any pictures at the water park - I thought we were going to be able to go again but the weather played a role in that decision.

Last weekend was the big state meet for Becca. We stayed at Chula Vista - a water park. There were 5 rides and I went down each one once. I think that we had to walk up three flights of stairs and I had to take a break on the way up, but the slides were so much FUN!! Especially the red one which was the fastest one there!! I wanted to go down many, many more times but I just couldn't do the stairs. Some of the rides I needed to have a tube with me. Katy was taking care of Raney so I said that I would grab the tubes and meet them upstairs for the big ride. I had to go down stairs to get the tubes (which I didn't know or I wouldn't have said I would get them) and then go up the 3 flights of stairs. Some young boy (maybe a freshman in HS) took the tubes and carried them upstairs for me and there was Raney and Katy - who also got tubes - waiting for me. My goal at the water park was to go down all the rides and I made that goal, but I really did want to go the next day and do all the rides again. However, it snowed and there was shoveling to do at home (preferably before it froze) so we left after the meet. That probably was good because I was more tired than I had realized.

The meet was good, but Becca hurt her Achilles tendon before it started so it was not her best, but I think that she had a good time. Hey, if nothing else we rode water slides!! I think that should be an annual thing. Otherwise this week has been quiet - just getting ready for the holidays.

Since it has been almost three weeks since my last spa day at Northwestern, I am feeling mostly myself this week. It's nice to have a visit from my old self. Tomorrow is treatment number 5 and then only one more. I can't believe the end is getting here for this part of the journey. I was hoping to be done tomorrow, but we will keep moving forward and trust that it will all be OK in the end.

I didn't walk yesterday. I think Kenosha got about 6-8 inches of snow and I needed to get brake work done on the car. The car wasn't stopping very well

- scary. So I was able to spend quality time with the Merlin people. Fun Fun Fun!!

I need to get the day started. I am off to the acupuncturist. I haven't been there in awhile. The weeks are getting away from me.
Hope the holiday season is off to a good start for all and that you stay nice and warm!!

I will chat later.

Posted Dec 10, 2007 10:40am

I just finished my walk - it is actually quite pleasant in Kenosha this morning (23 degrees) and with hot flashes I was warmer than last summer. I had to sport my baldness on my walk today and thought about my mom because as a mom I am always telling Raney and Becca to put on their hats and gloves and here I am taking them off.

Last Friday went well. Rob and I drove downtown and we were there about an hour and a half early for my genetic meeting to find out if I am mutated - which I am not. I don't have a gene that caused the cancer, so now I think that it is environmental or stress related. This takes a card off the table for my siblings, but my sisters and daughters are still put in a higher risk state.

We went over to American Girl to do some shopping (no telling the girls) with my sister. After that Rob ordered us a pizza for lunch and I went to check in. I was about 20 minutes early at this point and they took me right away and even drew my blood without the normal wait time. Jimee joined us and we heard about his honeymoon and saw a few pictures of Kristin and him surfing. If my brain works at the right time they might even get the wedding card that I have somewhere in this house - I can't remember where I put it.

I was put into a room and my numbers were good. My white counts were around 3.0 which is still a little low but high enough for Chemo!!!!
I will be thrilled to have this part of the journey done - not that I am looking forward to the rest, but my bones ache today and I am just tired.

58

After the spa (I was going to work on my Christmas cards but I fell asleep again) we went over to the Drake hotel for some soup and to look at their Christmas decorations - it was very nice. I love the city of Chicago.

The weekend was very quiet - we had nothing planned. We finished putting up the Christmas decorations and Raney and Becca played in the snow quite a bit. Rob cooked an Indian dish for us and we had friends join us for dinner. It was very relaxing. We have been watching almost all the Christmas

specials on ABC (I think that is the channel). I can't remember the last time I watched so much TV, but I am (was) very tired this weekend so I just let it be.

It was hard getting up this morning and I went to bed before the kids last night. Becca and Raney tracked me down for goodnight kisses. Sometimes it really does take everything I have to move and get the girls to school or wherever, but I do it because of the support and prayers that I get every day from you - so thank you!!!!

I better get going. I can't find my gloves at the moment and I know that I had them yesterday.

Have a wonderful week and sing Christmas carols all day long! Those songs put the singing into my kids so it is fun to listen to them.

Take care and Happy Holidays!!

Posted Dec 12, 2007 4:34pm

This week I have met my match and her name is Mother Nature!! Cancer doesn't stop me from walking (most days) but Mother Nature sure can put a wrench in my plans. Yesterday we had a "snow" day without any snow but it was icy, and today was even worse since the slush froze for my morning walk. A friend offered her treadmill and I think I am going to have to forego the outdoors and move my walk inside.

And the other thing about Mother Nature - this afternoon I heard birds singing, ice melting, sun shining and the temperature was actually very spring-like. I am not a fan of teasers! I want spring when it is spring! Spring-like weather in winter - that is like oil and water to me.

My legs hurt, especially my knees. I am hoping that this goes away soon because I can't get comfortable sitting or sleeping. I am taking pain pills for this and I handled the nausea better than this. I am really tired this week. I haven't been sleeping as well as I did last week, but I am going to give it a couple more days before calling the nurse to see what can be done. More pills are what she will offer and I might just take her up on it this time around.

Raney had to do a character description and she chose me. She counted the number of eyebrows and lashes that I have left because she had to describe what I look like, what I say, what I do, and how I make her feel. I am the craziest looking mom in her class. (For the moment.)

On the way to CCD today Becca asked if I was going to die. I said some day. She asked if the breast cancer was going to kill me. I told her that wasn't my plan so the rest of the car ride I heard the percentages that Raney and Becca are hoping that I don't die! One was 50/50. I spoke up on that one and said I wanted better odds. It then went to 1% for the cancer getting me. What a wonderful conversation I get to have with my children.

The other thing that I might be able to do that most moms can't do with their daughters is blossom! Raney and I may blossom together next year. Won't that be fun? Getting breasts together? Poor Raney - the joys of being the oldest.

I better get going; I hope everyone's holidays are stress-free and full of joy this year. I might even toast on New Year's for being chemo free. Join me in spirit (you can practice toasting now if you want).

LOL and LOL

Hello Friends

I did the treadmill today - walking by the lake with friends is a lot more fun but in Wisconsin I have to do what Mother Nature decides. I think we got about 8 inches this weekend.

Last week I went to a Christmas ornament exchange party. I picked a penguin with ruby glass slippers. He is very cute. A couple of my neighbors - who I see mostly in the summer - didn't recognize me in my hat. I am thinking it is more the lack of eyebrows that probably threw them off. I have one eyebrow that is not lying right and I am thinking of plucking it, but when you only have 4 it is hard to get rid of even the misbehaving hair. I just try to get it to lay correct - just like Harry Potter's hair. Afterwards I went out with a friend for an H2O martini. I was out until 9:30pm - a late night for me.

Saturday night, Rob grilled and started a pit fire. We then played Princess Monopoly and he won. You know how competitive boys are. It was a great night but I don't think that Rob will play that game again anytime soon. He was Mulan.

I still have my sleeping buddy. Raney pretends to cry if I try to give Becca a turn until she starts to sob for real. The actress in her is getting quite a workout. I have tried everything that I can think of to get her to sleep in her own bed, but she's in not budging. I am already telling her that she can't sleep with me after surgery, just so she is prepared.

We are getting ready for the holidays this week and hopefully I won't be wrapping on Christmas Eve like I usually do.

I don't think anything else exciting has been happening. I didn't walk last week because of the snow and ice. I had my walking buddies over for a breakfast instead. I served crepes with fruit, of course; I save the ice cream for my eating buddies (Raney and Becca). This is a nice alternative to walking, and much warmer.

I didn't sleep well last night (actually all last week has been hard to sleep) and I had something that I was going to share but now I can't remember; imagine that, my brain doesn't work. Only ONE more chemo left. I can't believe the end is almost here. I am staying downtown Thursday as my appointment is at 9:00am. I might go check out Macy's (aka Marshall Fields in the past) windows with my friend who is staying downtown with me.
I still get very tired and it is definitely more apparent this time around. I am nervous about the lack of energy with the kids off of school for the next two weeks.

Raney told me again how she doesn't have cancer but it is ruining her life. I can only imagine her life story! So I informed her on my thoughts of getting cancer and what I don't like about it. And that this is short-lived, even though it seems to be taking a long time. I know in the big picture that this is just a blink. I am grateful that there is chemo, radiation, and surgery available so I can lose my hair and get breasts. I will be the perkiest grandma in town at a ripe old age.

I need to get some things done so I will chat with you later.
Have fun getting ready for the holidays-

Talk to you later.

P.S. I started reading <u>Harry Potter</u> 3 again last night since I couldn't sleep. I don't get yelled at by Rob when he doesn't know I'm not sleeping. I just inform him in the morning!

Posted Dec 21, 2007 11:17am

I am writing as I am getting chemo - so therefore my numbers are good!!! I am 40 minutes in for my last spa day!!!!!!

I will let you go and I will catch up with you later this week.

Today is the solstice so we have a balance day, and tomorrow will be the start of getting longer days!!!! Summer here we come.

Happy Holidays, Merry Christmas, and thank you so much for your thoughts and prayers. I couldn't have done this without you!!!

May Santa bring you what you want.
LOL

Posted Dec 21, 2007 7:07pm

I don't have much time because Rob is cooking dinner, but I wanted to share with everyone: its official!!! NO MORE CHEMO!!!!!!! I was very nervous because I have a cold and I was afraid that my white counts were going to be low, but my blood work was the best it has been since I started this journey.

Thank you so much for your prayers. It is why I was able to get through chemo as well as I did!!!

Lots of love and many thanks.

Merry Christmas and here's to a rocking '08!!!!!
P.S. I will write about my week so stay posted.

Posted Dec 26, 2007 9:36pm

Merry Christmas a bit late. Since it has been awhile since I last updated I am going to skip last week - just know that I made it through the final days before Christmas without too many problems.

One thing I will share is that I am going to write a book, *How to do Holidays on Chemo.* Each person's gifts are wrapped on different days and with different color wrapping paper. As I was wrapping for Raney and Becca, I wrote their names on the box to help me out. I thought that was good enough, but nope, after I put on the wrapping paper not only did I forget what was in the box, but I couldn't remember whose gift it was. Becca (who still believes in Santa) saw Raney's name written on a box that she opened from Santa and said, "Oops Santa must have gotten confused." Little did she know how true that statement was! And Raney ended up with both pairs of PJs and the stuffed animals. Try to explain that one without spilling the beans. How confused can Santa be? When I was telling my brother Ryan that I was going to assign different colors I said Rob will get blue and Becca will get blue...that was enough to get the jokes going! But when Becca and Raney were younger, Raney was given pink clothes and Becca was given blue clothes so there really was a reason for Becca to get blue wrapping paper. And Rob, of course, was given blue because he is a boy - but I changed him to purple. I saved the book, but Ryan is not getting anything for Christmas next year!

Christmas Eve was a very nice time. I put make-up on for the big day and I thought that I looked scary. Raney and Becca put on mascara and I said that I didn't think that I would put any on the 4 lashes that I have left (and I still have one eyebrow left on the left side so we will see if I get out of chemo with a brow and a lash). We went into Chicago to Rob's 2nd cousins'. They had just had a baby about 6 months ago, baby Henry. It's hard to remember those days, but then again it's hard to remember anything these days.

Even though I had everything wrapped early this year (first time ever!!!), I still was up I think until 1:00am so when Raney woke up around 5:45 I lied and told her that it was only 4 and to go back to bed. She woke up again around 6:15. I tried to lie again but she was smarter this time. It took her about 4 times of coming upstairs every 15 minutes before I could get out of bed, around 7:15. Better than last year when we got up at 5:30am. Family started showing up around 1ish. I wasn't feeling my best but as people showed up I felt better and better (but still very tired). Katy had said that about me; I get energy from people. It must be true because I was up until 11 on Christmas. Our day was packed with people, food, and crazy gifts. It was a good time.

Christmas felt different this year for many reasons, but of course one is the cancer changes a lot with me. My eyes have been opened to a love in this world that is so much more than I realized. Not that I didn't know it existed - it just is even more. I woke up today (after sleeping through the night) totally recharged mentally; my body on the other hand is extremely tired. I felt like I was on cloud nine. What a wonderful gift to have. I just hope that I can keep that feeling alive in me for the rest of my days.

Today was another great day. Some of my family stayed at a hotel down the street (Raney and Becca stayed the night and are there again) so they will come back for lunch. We pulled out a game, started dinner, and then the wine was opened. We just ate, drank, and hung out. I even had a glass of wine. I am a homebody who likes to have people over. That's the perfect day for me.

I have more to say but I am too tired to write so I will chat later
Sweet dreams

P.S. This chemo messes with the nails and I am hoping that I won't lose my big toe nail, but I think that I am losing that battle. I can always paint a nail on.

Posted Jan 1, 2008 9:09pm

An FYI for now - I sent the kids to bed at 8:20 this evening and Raney just came downstairs. It was too good to be true. I will update on my New Year's later.

I have been thinking of all of you, and I toasted you for all that you have done for me. HAPPY NEW YEAR!! I am so grateful to all of you, and there is no way I can ever thank you enough for all your kindness.

I did also want to let you know that I learned that I could put captions on the photos. I did that and I will post new photos tomorrow. I tried tonight but the server couldn't be found. I guess it is taking the day off.

I better go back to being a mom and not an author for the time. I guess I will just stay upstairs so Raney will go to sleep.

Love to all and I pray that 2008 is a rocking year. I have faith that wonderful things are going to happen this year!!!!

Today was the first day back to school and I did not want to wake up. I slept on/off from about 2:00am until the sweet sound of my alarm clock at 6:30am. (Tonight I am sleeping with a hammer and I will feel GREAT when I smash the alarm tomorrow!!) I hit snooze which puts Raney and Becca behind schedule. I know that is a bad thing but I am tired, so snooze gets hit and hit again. When I finally left it alone, I was taunted by (I am not sure who sings this song) "your body is a wonderland" and then something to the effect of "your hair around your face..." Yeah - what a way for the baldy, and soon to be boobless (now there is a wonderland), lady who didn't sleep and has to get her kids out the door for the first time in 12 days to have to listen to because she is already 15 minutes later than she should be (and yes, I typed that all in one breath). The girls made it to school on time. Now granted, breakfast was eaten in the car and Becca was putting her socks on in the car, but they were on time.

I was going to write this last year - doesn't 2007 seem a lifetime ago already? - but here are my thoughts today.

I have had people mention to me forgetting about 2007 and wasn't it a bad year. And while I would not freely choose this path that was chosen for me, I can't say that I regret it either. I don't know what is in store for me, and I am terrified that the surgeon might come back and say something that I don't want to hear (that has happened before and I try not to have fear but I am human), but this path has shown so much beauty that I wouldn't change it now. I have heard from people that I haven't spoken to in years; I have people that I haven't met sending me care packages; and friends, neighbors, and family carrying me through every step of this journey. That I believe strongly, makes planet Earth a better place for all mankind. Every act of kindness ripples to unknown numbers of people. How can I say that this is a "bad" path? I have such gratitude and thankfulness for all of you. I just feel I don't really show it to the fullest extent, but I pray that you all understand and believe I truly am grateful for everything: every meal, every kind word, every ride for the kids, every card, every prayer...and of course every bottle of wine (I drink a little now). Who knew that I could be so sappy? (No, I haven't had a glass of wine today, but after calling the

66

insurance company, the doctor's office, and I can't remember who else, I have thought about it.)

I will have to update you on my New Year's later. I have new pictures to post but I need to get Raney from Girl Scouts.

Again, to 2008: a year to embrace because the beginning is going to be very hard for me. Losing boobies (not as funny anymore) but I am going to have a party to say "goodbye to the ladies" a couple of nights before surgery. I was going to go topless but I think I will keep the shirt on! Maybe I will go braless and let the ladies fly free. Or I could burn my bras since I won't need them again. That could be fun, right? The possibilities are endless...

Have a great day and talk to you soon!

Posted Jan 8, 2008 9:59am

Today is my baby's golden birthday. Hard to believe she is 8. She wanted to know what time she was born this morning. I wonder if she is going to share that information with someone in her class. Her birthday treats are rice krispies, simple to make and delicious but I messed up the first batch. I burned the butter and added the marshmallows before I saw the burnt butter so I wasn't able to make 2 batches so none for me - bummer!!! I guess cooking and (now I can say this) the side effects of chemo don't mix - probably for at least a year!? My brain is still slow and it is so annoying!!

New Year's was nice. We went to Lake Geneva and, because of the weather, only my cousin and his wife made it up for a visit. It was nice to have a glass of the bubbly (or two, but who's counting?). The only problem was my brother was supposed to bring dessert, and since he didn't make it we went to a local store to get some ice cream. Luckily, we had part of the main dinner in our oven so we had food, and lots of it. Becca and I made it past midnight. Raney woke up around 1am mad because she thought I had moved her to the couch - she didn't realize she'd fallen asleep there and I just left her. I was hoping that she would sleep until morning, but I should have known better.

There is a lot that I should know better, but I tell you this brain! Maybe instead of a boob job I can ask for a brain job. The kids went to Lake Geneva with these pink glitter ballet type shoes and we had about 5 inches of snow. A friend wanted them to go sledding. I don't know what I was thinking. I mean, when in Wisconsin do you not need winter clothes at the beginning of January? I guess it's better not to have a brain in the winter so my kids don't fry like a lobster in the summer, but then some school projects aren't turned in on time. It is such a no-win battle! My advice is to play Sudoku and keep your mind working. A brain is a terrible thing to lose.

OK, now on to the big news: surgery is set for January 21 at the new Prentice hospital in Chicago (by Watertower). I might get a lake view room with a 42 inch plasma TV. I might want to stay a month with those accommodations! And I get to order food whenever!! Talk about feeling like a queen - a queen with BOOBS!! I misunderstood the surgeon when he said no reconstruction before radiation. No reconstruction with tissue involved before radiation. What I will wake up with is temporary saline implants that have a port so that saline can be added until the desired size is attained. The possibilities!! But since every time I want to add a size I have to go to Chicago, let's just say an A cup will be just fine. I am thrilled to know that I am not going to wake up looking like a boy, but I am going to lose - here are the gory details - my nipples until - a silver lining in every cloud - my implants become permanent and then not only do I get my nipples back, but I get tattoos. The possibilities are endless. I don't know about the surgeon's opinion on fun tattoos, but it keeps me amused. A benefit to a simple mind - easily amused.

I am running out of time so let me finish the details. To my knowledge my surgery will be around 3:00pm Monday and I will be released on Thursday. My sister, Raney, and Becca are going to stay in Chicago, so the girls are able to visit a few times. Raney is nervous about the IV and the machines, so if anyone has any experience of how to help prepare them please share. Thanks. On Jan 29th I start the process of radiation. I will have 33 treatments Monday - Friday at Lake Forest Hospital. I am not sure of the exact date that radiation starts because I think that I go about 3-4 times to get set up before the actual treatment starts. If I start by Feb 11th I will finish with half our spring break left. That would be cool.

I am out of time and I don't want to lose this update.
Have a wonderful day and talk to you later.

Posted Jan 8, 2008 10:26am

I forgot to mention that for Christmas my brother-in-law (my drinking buddy) gave us a case of wine - just kidding - he gave us tickets to go see *Wicked* at the Oriental in downtown Chicago. It was a great play. If you have a chance to see it I highly recommend it. The singing just blows me away. I read the book as well and the play is adapted but there are some differences. Raney and Becca really liked it as well and want to see it again.

I haven't been walking every day but I am doing OK. I am using a friend's treadmill because even with 60 degrees I am not able to go outside with the rain and tornados that Kenosha has been getting. Hopefully, I will get a couple of outside walking days before surgery.

Until the next time.

Posted Jan 16, 2008 5:37pm

Well the countdown has begun - actually I have been counting down since July 27th, but I wasn't sure what date to count down to so at least now I have an end date. I remember thinking (back in the day when my brain actually functioned) when the doctor told me that I had breast cancer, "CUT IT OUT!!! I DON'T WANT IT IN MY BODY!!! WHO CARES ABOUT THE BREASTS-TAKE THEM OFF". Now that I have a date and I am losing my breasts (getting fake ones though so no flatness!!!) I am not so sure how I feel about this. I have mixed emotions. I want my evil friend to lose his home, but I am not sure I like the way his home is being destroyed. I know that it is a better way to survive and that is my goal. So the feeble brain that I have gets that reason for the operation, but the emotional part of me is freaking out.

69

That is the way of women - we are such complex individuals; never a dull moment in our brains. I feel like I should have the house in order, almost like I need to 'nest'. And with the cravings that I have one could almost believe that I am pregnant instead of a cancer person. I can't say patient because I still don't feel like one. Maybe after surgery when I look at myself - no hair, no eyebrows, no lashes, and no real boobs - I will either feel like a patient or maybe a droid that belongs on the Terminator Show. I am transforming, but into what? That is the big question of the day.

Sometimes when I look into the mirror I see myself, but other times I have no idea who is looking back at me.

We have a great plan for Raney and Becca. My sister is keeping them downtown Monday - Wednesday night. We will return to Kenosha on Thursday. This way my children will get to see the great room that I am staying in - I keep calling my room a hotel because I get to order food whenever I want, and have a great, big plasma TV. I may not want to leave for awhile.

Raney is hounding me for the computer, so I need to let you go.

I hope to chat one more time before I go through my transformation. I think this would be so much easier if it was elective, but it is what it is.

Keep on truckin'

Posted Jan 17, 2008 12:47pm

I remember awhile ago my brother-in-law wrote about what other parties I would be having during this journey. I was going to have a "goodbye to the ladies" party with sparkling wine, of course, and breast shaped cakes (with a Hershey kiss on top), pinning the boobies on the lady, and reading from Judy Blume's book, *Are you there, God? It's me, Margaret* - a must read for girls in 4-5th grade. I hadn't really thought about what food to serve but I am running out of time to fit all that I want to do before the big (or should we call it the reduction?) event. But it has been fun talking about it. I might have a "welcome to the new ladies" party when I am feeling better (off pain

70

medication so I can have bubbly). Who knows? I like parties and this journey has given me many different types of parties. I am special!!!! I can be vain for the day.

I need to get some things done so I can party with my sister for her birthday on Sunday.

Have a great day

My surgery is scheduled for 2:30pm on Monday. I need to sign in at 1:00pm. I can't eat after midnight (there goes my planned midnight run to the refrigerator - I thought that I would be able to eat up to about 3:00am) and no liquids after 8:00am. Surgery is supposed to be about 4.5 hours with two surgeons. I am not sure how long the first surgeon will take, but once Dr. Bethke is done, he will come out and talk to the family and then Dr. Fine will be putting in my temporary implants.

I met with someone today who still has her temporary implants - she let me feel them; hard as a rock, but no sagging!!! I didn't realize that they would be hard. She seemed to be doing well with them. I am hoping that I will have no problems with saline so I don't have to do any tissue reconstruction. I would like fewer surgeries if possible. She said that it took her a month before she was comfortable driving. I am hoping to be able to drive pretty soon after surgery; however that would eliminate grocery shopping, so maybe I won't rush it.

I need to get Raney from school so I have to go but I wanted to let you know when I am going to have the body redesigned. I hope that I like it when it is all done. Nothing I would have done on my own but it is what it is. At least there are researchers who have learned how to work with the cancer to make it livable. I just want it out there that I thank each and every researcher and person who went through cancer before me so I will be able to stick around and be a hot (old) Grandma.

If I don't have a chance to talk before Monday, my brother will be updating on the pages for me so you don't have to wait for me to feel up to typing on the computer.

Thanks for your support and prayers. The next phase is upon us and we move forward!!!!
Happy Birthday, Baby Sister!!!

This is a test. I wanted to make sure that I could post an update for Patty. I will not guarantee that my spelling will be any better than Patty's, and she had the "chemo-brain" excuse!

Patty also asked that I keep the updates funny; I will do my best, but while Patty may have lost her hair and her eyebrows, I am only losing my hair, so I will not be as funny as she.

Patty knows how to use a good teacher, and our mom was one of the best. Mom showed all of us strength and courage when dealing with serious issues. Patty has taken those lessons and with the use of this CarePage has been able to share them with all of us.

Patty will be updating her page as soon as she is able, and until then I will do my best to provide you with updates on the progress that she will be making.
Jimee

Well, the countdown has begun. After midnight there is to be nothing, not even water, until I am back in the room - which I am guessing will be around 8:30pm. No one is going to want to visit me until after I have eaten something! I will be so hungry and thirsty I won't care that I have fake ones.

Today I went to my niece's to celebrate my sister's birthday. All my brothers and most of my sisters and half my sisters-in-law were there. It was a very nice time, but a short visit. The kids have school tomorrow so we had to get home at a decent time. I had a couple of friends stop by for some bubbly and to toast to a whole new healthier path. We finished the bottle - so I am off to quite a healthy beginning. Bubbly is such a happy drink. I should drink it more often.

I am a bit nervous but I think I will be OK. Today was the day that I really could have used my mom, but I know she will be watching the surgeons tomorrow. However, just a hug from her would be really great today.

I had lots of hugs from family and friends and people called to wish me well. I am so grateful for all of you. As the priest said today at mass, we are all lambs of God.
So baa baa! I need to get some beauty sleep.

Until I can get back on line I am handing over the reins to Jimee.
Love to all

Posted Jan 21, 2008 5:48pm

THE EVIL FRIEND IS GONE!!!!!

Patty, Rob, and the girls arrived at the hospital early and met Dad, Eileen, Linda, Katy, and me. Patty was taken to pre-op at 1:14 p.m. (Which for those of you who do not know, is our mom's birthday). At 3:36p.m. she went into surgery. About 5:00p.m. the nurse came to talk to Rob, to tell him that the evil friend is out. Patty has about another hour to remove the other side, and then the reconstruction begins. Patty will have about an hour in recovery, and then we can see her.

Patty promised that she would not be modest for the surgeons!
I will post another when we have more updates.
Jimee

It is 7:00 pm and Dr. Bethke just spoke to Rob. In his words, everything was "routine" - at least for him, not so much for the family. Patty is now with Dr. Fine. That should be about 1 - 1 1/2 hours.

Patty should get the pathology report on Wednesday.

Dr. Bethke also said that she might be able to go home on Wednesday.

Everything is going according to plan.

THE EVIL FRIEND HAS BEEN EVICTED!!!!!!!!!!!!!!!!!!!!

Now there were none. Dr. Fine just left, and, of course, Patty did wonderful. She is going to laugh when she finds out that her doctor referred to her as a pair of old jeans. He said everything went fine. He said there were a few thin spots (totally normal) and he had to put in an internal patch, like you would put a patch on a pair of jeans. She will be in recovery for an hour or so. Dr. Fine also said that he would expect that she will be sent home on Wednesday.

Patty has two drains, one on the left and one on the right. She also has internal pain management, which will reduce her need for pain medicine.

NO MORE EVIL FRIEND!!!!!!!!!!!!!!!!!!!!

It is 10:36p.m. and Patty is in her room, 1488. She is awake and said hello to the entire group: Rob, Eileen, Katy, Dad, Kristin and me. Rob asked her if she got her ice chips, and she said, "Yes, and I am not giving them back."

Another hurdle successfully behind her.
Jimee

Good morning from Northwestern Hospital.

Patty and Rob both had a restful evening. Patty was sitting in the chair for awhile this morning. She is currently watching a big screen TV, showing restful, scenic images.
Jimee

It is 5:50p.m. and Patty has walked down the hall and is sitting in the waiting room with our dad. Linda went in Patty's room to pick up some coats, and the nurse went in looking for Patty. The nurse has found her, and is giving her the good stuff.

Jimee

Patty is saying goodnight to the girls. She says that she is doing better, but she is not done, and she is asking you to keep up with the prayers.

She is going to have a blood test in the morning and she will then find out if she will be released.

Jimee

Patty has figured out the drug thing and her body was ready to go home. She is now sitting on her couch in Kenosha. She was discharged around 11:30a.m. She is currently under the care of a babysitter (her neighbor Beth); Rob went to the pharmacy to pick up her meds.

Soon, she will have the strength to do this herself, just like everything else.

Jimee

It is Tuesday at about 9:45am and Patty's fever finally broke. She decided that having her chest removed, and an expander device (which hurts like hell) put in its place, was not enough. She decided that getting the flu was the next thing on her agenda. That is why she has not been updating; she has been sleeping, trying to recover. Good news from Patty is that her fever is gone and she is still alive and kicking. The girls have gone back to school and Aunt Katy has been staying at Patty's to help out. Patty has 3 drains and they are working well. Hopefully with her strength improving, she can begin to add to the blog.

It is now 5:15p.m. and Patty and Rob are on the way home from a visit with Dr. Fine. The nurse wanted Patty to come in since the fever came back. It is still the flu; the good news is that they removed the drains. Patty had 3 drains for fluid removal. Her next trip to the doctor is next week.

Jimee

Someone told me that Jimee was brief and I finally read his update - and yes he is brief. It must be the lawyer in him.

Thank you, Jimee, for those exciting updates. You sure put the people on the edge of their chairs waiting for the next update! I don't think Jimee is comfortable sharing the gory details.

But let's update for a moment before we back track. Yesterday was the first day since Jan 25th that I didn't spend most of the day sleeping. The flu really put me on my *** - more than the chemo. I feel like I have really been out of touch, but I have two days in a row awake and I even laughed yesterday, but I will get to that.

Back to what I remember of the surgery: that would be nothing - thank God!!!! I do remember seeing my family after getting back to the room. My surgery lasted about an hour longer than we were told (but they did take me about an hour later then they said). Supposedly my explanation was that they were missing a scalpel. I don't remember saying this and I can't get an answer that would explain why I would have told my family this. What I do remember telling them is that a truck ran me over. Surgery hurts like hell (sorry for the lack of grating, but that is one pain that I can't imagine ever forgetting). I had the kindest nurse come in every 2 (or maybe 4?) hours and drug me up. The motto 'Say No to Drugs' doesn't exist in a hospital. It's more like, 'Say Yes, a LOT!!!'

Tuesday morning I woke up around 7:30am (they do say no to sleeping at a hospital). I was told that I could go home that morning. I wasn't sure how I was going to get in a car. I went to the bathroom and was sitting in a chair by 9:30am. Rob and the girls had just come back from breakfast when I started to react to the anesthesia. The nurse called the resurrection team; they called a code red. I never passed out, but Rob and my sister watched 5-6 people run down the hallway to my room with a crash cart with paddles. The thought of them using paddles hurts my chest still. That got me another day in the hospital. I would not have been able to truly enjoy the big screen if they sent me home less than 12 hours after surgery, since most my time was spent sleeping.

Rob and I left on Wednesday. Jimee told me that we didn't call anyone to let them know that we were leaving but I can't remember - I was on some good drugs. I am sure that I would have told Katy because she had Raney and Becca. Wednesday and Thursday were uneventful. I took naps but I think I was feeling OK, then Friday came and all hell broke loose. I had a temperature from Jan 25 through the 30. This is a problem after surgery because I didn't know that I had the flu until Monday, so there was the fear of an infection. My sister, Katy, said that I was incoherent at one point in talking with a doctor and she was shocked that they didn't have me go to the ER, but maybe because the fever would go down with Advil?

The doctors were not too worried. I don't know.

But on Tuesday the plastic surgeon's office had me go downtown in the afternoon so we got the girls out of school and left at 2:15pm. We made it downtown by 3:30pm (unbelievable timing). Too bad it isn't that easy to always get downtown, but all it ended up being was the flu. The trip was not all lost because they did take out the tubes. And they were gross to me so I was happy to see them go. They didn't hurt - just gross. They didn't bother Raney and Becca though, so that is a good thing; no nightmares about Mommy turning into something else.

I am going to sign off for now and I will finish my update tomorrow when you get to read about how Becca feels about the new boobs.

Sleep well and talk to you soon

It is good to be back in the saddle - and thank you, Jimee, I needed someone to keep posting until I felt better. Thanks for all the prayers and thoughts. Love to all

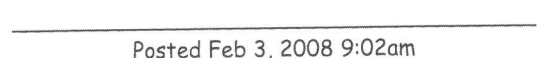

Posted Feb 3, 2008 9:02am

Rob and the girls are off to get my next nurse, Jimee; my last one got away from me. Katy ran out the open door - not looking back once. (It wasn't that bad, but I think I did see a huge smile as she drove away singing - I am free! I am free!).

Poor Katy; not only didn't she get much notice on the additional days of taking care of me, she also endured two snow days with both Rob working out of the house and the kids at home. One day was -26 wind chill so Raney and

Becca couldn't go outside. The second day the kids were outside but ringing the doorbell - which made the dog bark - which made Rob yelled because he was on a work call; it was like bad reality TV because this must have happened at least 4 times. That was the day that I started to laugh again. Sometimes I just find the domino effect very funny - the only problem with that is, ouch!! It hurts to laugh - or get scared.

We tried to watch a scary movie and the first time I jumped we had to turn it off because, ouch!!

While Raney and Becca were outside, Katy and I played *Disney Scene It* with no clues like we had given the girls. There was a tie-breaker at one point in the game. The person with the longest hair won the tie-breaker. I thought that was truly unfair, but Katy took the win anyways. She is not the type of nurse to let the patient win.

When Katy was here, she kept Raney company so that I didn't have to worry about Raney trying to sneak into bed with me. Raney is a mover while she sleeps, and I can't have her swinging her arms on me. I have been hit in the chest area a couple of times and OUCH.

Last night as I was getting ready for bed, I left Raney in her room with fake tears. I got out of the bathroom and Raney had gotten out of her bed and made the Wall of China in the middle of my bed so that she wouldn't touch me. Brownie points for coming up with a solution. Every time I move in bed, it hurts and Raney kept asking, "Are you OK, mom?" I will be looking forward to that pain being something in the past. I didn't ask the plastic surgeon how much it hurts to get new boobs - I am not sure I would have been brave enough to do this if I knew the truth. The implants go under the muscles. There will not be much pumping up because that sounds painful. I have at least 6 months of the temporary ones and then another surgery - I should have thought about that as well.

I think that updates the week that I was down and out. I almost forgot one more update. I lost my big toenail last night. Becca wanted to keep it in a plastic bag - GROSS.

Now onto the update you all have been waiting for: the boob update.

I told my sister that they are ugly, and I still think they are ugly. My sister said that $10,000 boobs aren't ugly. What I need to think when I look at them is that they are a work in process. They are not as bad as I feared - but there will be no going topless in Mexico until the plastic surgeon does a lot more magic on them.

It is a strange feeling though; my skin is covering the implants, but they don't feel real. Maybe when this is all said and done, I can go back feeling like they are mine. Right now they are blobs, but they don't sag like the old ones. I actually have some cleavage so I am not flat. I told Rob that I won't need to buy any more bras so I can save $hundreds over my lifetime - but I am going to buy at least one useless bra from Victoria Secret.

My sweet little child told me, "No offense, mommy, but those don't look so good on you." The truth of a child; gotta love it. At least it seems that Raney and Becca are not phased by the fake boob thing at all. I know that they were glad to have Aunt Katy around for a week and a half, but I think that they were getting tired of me sleeping the week away. I am so glad the flu is over.

I am going to have some breakfast and enjoy the peace and quiet until my next nurse is on duty. My sister-in-law took the train, so she has an exit date already scheduled.

Have a great day!

Posted Feb 3, 2008 12:10pm

My bad--I forget to share the pathology report-oops...
3 tumors were found in the left breast
5.2 cm
1.0 cm
0.2 cm and the tumors were 4 mm away from the chest wall. There are some tests that came back negative (which is positive) but I can't remember what the tests tell the doctor.
And 7 lymph nodes were removed and all 7 tested positive for cancer.
The right breast and the lymph nodes are all clean. Yeah for the right!!!!

What this means is that I will be radiated 28 times in the chest and neck area.
I go back to the radiologist Feb. 11, so I think I will start radiation Feb. 14 and finish the Monday of our spring break. Dr. Imperato says there should be no problems with eating or nausea with radiation. I guess I'll just be more tired toward the end and the skin area will look and feel like a bad sunburn.

I see the plastic surgeon Feb. 5 and the surgeon Feb. 12.

Enjoy the Superbowl -

Have a great day

Posted Feb 6, 2008 9:34am

Well, we didn't get the 20 inches of snow that was promised so my kids had to get up and go to school. Raney was up by 5:45am hoping for that snow day.

I saw the plastic surgeon (Dr. Fine) yesterday and he said that I am healing nicely. He wouldn't do any more pumping up because of radiation; he said that I could come back a month after radiation when I am feeling better. He was kind enough to share with me that I won't be feeling that great during radiation, but I should have no problems eating, even with being radiated around the neck area. I did ask him about the patch that Jimee had written about; it came from the refrigerator. I didn't ask if it was someone else's skin. It's better sometimes not to hear the obvious.

I also received a letter from the radiologist. He described me as a thin, frail, young woman! Frail, please! Frail people don't go around kicking cancer butt (I learned the a-s-s word is not allowed in Carepages blogs) and I am kicking cancer butt because I never want to do this again! Even though I still have enough support and love to probably do this for the next ninety years, I would rather be cancer free.

OK, enough about the doctor visits and letters. I went out of the house this week!!!! I went to a friends' on Super bowl as my first non-doctor outing. On

81

Monday, I went grocery shopping with my sister-in-law, and then we did a little shopping at Marshalls. Yesterday, after going downtown, we went out to lunch and then to the outlet mall before the kids came home from school. Today, we will hang out at home due to the weather - they are still predicting up to 20 inches of snow - but as Becca said, we are by the lake, so we may only get 5 inches. We had to talk about how the weather people predicate the weather for about a half hour after bedtime - so Becca didn't want to move too quickly this morning.

I am feeling a bit disorganized in my blogging today; sorry.

I have gone to this place in Northbrook a couple of times called, The Cancer Wellness Center. All the services are free for cancer patients and their families. I would go a lot more if it was closer - their services are great. They are having a walk/run in April that Raney has the family signed up for. She also created a team to help raise funds. We are called *Bosom Buddies*. We (all 4 of us) are doing the 5k walk, but Raney and Becca want to run it, so I am trying to get my brother, Jimee, and his wife, Kristin, to run with the girls. Raney sent out an email to the people that I had emails for to ask for help in reaching her $2,500 goal. If you are interested in joining us for the walk/run it is at Independence Grove, Libertyville, IL April 27. You can check out the website @ cancerwellness.org for all the details. Or if you would like to donate, that also can be done online. Raney is going to be written up in their newsletter.

I am sure that these things help her deal with the cancer that has invaded our lives. I try to keep us as normal as possible. That really isn't possible, but we try anyways. Just such a bad time (as if there is a good time to get cancer) for all that Raney and Becca will be going through anyway (being girls), and then Mommy getting cancer on top of all that. They are going to know that women are tough and nothing will keep us down. WE ARE WOMEN! HEAR US ROAR! (And my kids have the roaring down.)

I am running out of time before I get logged off so I will say goodbye. I am watching my nurse shovel snow for me. My nurses are paid poorly and have new job responsibilities thrown at them at will. Who would like to be my nurse for the next week? It's fun up to be up at 6:30am and in bed by

8:30pm with lots of variety during the day. Please submit your resume, if you are interested.

Have a great day.

I was back at the doctor's again today; for Becca, not me. She has strep again!! 5th time in about 11 months. We are now on the watch of too many strep infections in a season. If this continues, she will have to see a nose, throat, and ear specialist, and then maybe the removal of her tonsils. I think that I have enough white blood cells that I will not get strep; I am just hoping Raney doesn't get it again.

I have been getting out every day. Even 18 inches of snow didn't stop me from climbing into the car and being chauffeured around town. I will like it when I can walk outside again; I miss the walks down by the lake. I, along with many others, am ready for spring to arrive.

Monday, I will know my radiation schedule, and then the light at the end of the tunnel will be light (even though I know that for the next 5 years I will be visiting all my doctor Friends, but that will just be follow ups).

I am able to move my arms more every day but it is amazing how little I can move them since surgery. I keep stretching every day. I tried a broom exercise, but didn't do so well with that one yet. I am hoping that I will be able to play tennis by summertime (which will be a real miracle, seeing that I didn't play tennis before).

Well, lunch is ready, so I am going to eat--

Have a wonderful day and I will chat with you later.

Hello Everyone,

I went to see the surgeon today. I am doing fine and will need to see him again in 6 months. I will then go once a year for the next five years to see him. He gave me a complete copy of my pathology report and I now know more about my breasts then I ever thought possible. I know the weight and the area of the tissue and something called skin ellipse and other things; more information than the common woman knows or wants to know about her breasts. And to think, all we used to care was if they were going to be bigger than a B cup!

Remember, Ladies, the good old days of getting them? Fighting with our moms because of the hormones, and being either really embarrassed or really excited because we were becoming women or the first bra shopping trip - who could forget?

Let me share a secret about the fake ones: getting fake ones HURTS like hell. It shouldn't be so bad, seeing what I had to go through the first time around when I was younger. I paid my dues then. That is not to be the case the second time around. I try to make them wiggle or move and they don't. I wondered today if I will be watching woman for the rest of my lives to see if theirs move. I might be slightly jealous, until I go to the old people home! When others' move it proves they are real, and mine don't move so I am therefore fake. I am hoping once they are done and the plastic surgeon does his magic, I will like them more. Dr. Fine used a word that I can't remember right now, but he sounded confident that they are going to turn out ok. 'Contour' that is the word he used. I am going to be contoured in 6-8 months. Doesn't that sound fun!!! I am going to get a shirt that states "I have been contoured!! Have you?"

Yesterday I went and saw the radiologist. I start radiation Monday 2/18 for 28 times. I had to reach over my head and hold on to handles as they put me through a scanner. That hurt, but it probably did my arm good to have to stretch like that for about 20 minutes. I also got 3 tattoos; look at me, living on the edge! They are very boring - just three blue dots. I didn't have a choice about my color, but they are still tattoos. I have always wanted a tattoo but never got around to getting one. The left side I didn't even feel - I am numb on that side and the upper part of my left arm has some numbing to it. I have been told it won't be as numb for the rest of my life but that there always is some numbing.

I finally got the lymph node thing. Dr Bethke only had to explain it to me about 3-4 times. I would never have made medical school for even a day. Because all seven of my lymph nodes came back positive for cancer I will be radiated in the neck area (I don't remember the medical name for it) because there are lymph nodes there, but Dr. Bethke stated that he could not feel cancer in them so there was no point in removing them. Removing them doesn't help with the survival rate and it puts me at a higher risk for swelling of the arm.

Here's for my doctor friends who read the blog-
estrogen receptor positive 100%
progesterone receptor low positive 10%
p53 10% positive - I have no idea what this is
HER-2/neu 0% score 0 negative - which I think is a good thing.

I am not sure when I am going to see the oncologist again but I think that it will be in a couple of weeks, if not sooner.

I am very backwards today-
I went to a play on Saturday with Jimee, Raney and a friend of Raney's - Becca stayed home with Rob because she wasn't feeling that well yet, but she is better now and she tries to boss me as soon as she gets home from school. January baby - what was I thinking!!! The play was *Tom Sawyer* and it was at a small theatre in Racine. Sunday I think that I stayed inside due to the negative wind chill factor.

I am getting better every day, and I thank you for all your thoughts and prayers. Please keep up the good work because it is working.

I hope you are enjoying the winter weather and have a wonderful week.
Love to all

I hit a wrong button, and my message erased – bummer, it was my funniest yet.

I went to my card making class last night and my sweetum was waiting up for me when I got home at 9:30; not Rob, but Raney. I am not sure she knows how to sleep without me in the house. Someday, maybe.

Today I did a few errands to get ready for Valentine's Day. I also went back to work at my book keeping job, but I did have my co-worker to help out and do my filing for me. I am not sure that my arms are ready for that type of stretching. I will be happy when my arms are somewhat back to normal.
I thought about taking up running since I won't be bouncing anymore in my life. I keep trying and they don't move. Tennis and running - I am going to be in the best shape of my life when I am able to move my arms again.
I am going to sign off and hang out with Raney - Becca is at gymnastics.

Have a great night.
Love to all

Time to update again. Since we last spoke, I have been put on tamoxifen. This is the pill that I might have to take up to five years. Because of my age & the extent of my cancer (7 lymph nodes) I started the pill before radiation. They normally like to wait until after radiation because I guess it will make the radiation affect the skin more, but they wanted me to start the medicine right away.

My side effects are fun for the whole family - more intense hot flashes, because the other ones weren't hot enough or often enough, and mood swings (what family doesn't love those?). If you see me chasing the kids down the street naked just chalk it up to a mood swing and a hot flash; no need to call anyone...

I started radiation on Tuesday. Monday was a planning session. I had to have my arms above my head for about 40 minutes on Monday, and that was a LOT of pain. My arms don't move that way yet. Yesterday I thought radiation was supposed to be quick and painless. Well the radiation part might be, but lying with my arms over my head for about 20 minutes at this time is not painless. They couldn't get the right angle because my arms are not cooperating quite yet. The last two nights I had to take 4 Tylenols to get to sleep. They keep promising me that the next one will be shorter, but we didn't get there yet.

Today's day - where do I begin? The girls were fine and we even got to school on time (they have been late about 7-8 times this year and that is a lot for us) and I stopped to fill up the tank in my van. I need to back up here. I started driving again on Monday, Feb. 18th. My car sat in the driveway last week because my dad was the chauffer and he prefers his car. Today I took my car to school and stopped for gas on the way home and there was a terrible smell from the engine. So what does every female do when it comes to car engines? I popped the hood and checked the transmission and brake fluid; both were fine by the way. I go in to pay for the gas (they have old pumps) and I ask how can I check my antifreeze fluid. The lady behind the desk asks me why I think it is antifreeze – um, because I checked the other fluids. I think that is the only other fluid in an engine (that might be wrong). I think I impressed her with my vast knowledge of the engine. I drove it up to the garage and the mechanic verified that something is leaking and it is probably the antifreeze. See how smart I am?? Luckily my dad was here and we took his car to my 2nd out of 28 radiation treatments--only to hear those dreaded words "the machine is down for the day. We will tack on the treatment on the end." Which means at this rate I will be finished on April Fool's Day. Maybe that will be a good day to finish! Last's years fool's day did my brother Jimee good (he got engaged on that day).

Other than my arms hurting all the time and my radiation treatments getting delayed a day (they did warn me that this might happen), everything else is OK. With the rest of the Midwest, I am really ready for grilling weather and warm sun rays upon my face. That alone will lift my spirits and I can get out and walk again. I am running out of ideas for cooking inside. We grill as much as we can outside until the d@$#% bitter cold hits and we have to cook inside for days on end. Then with all the snow I can't get to the grill, even if I wanted to today.

I think that I am a bit crabby today - I want radiation to get going everyday so that I can shut the door on that chapter and I want my arms to stop hurting. I am going to go to rehabilitation at Lake Forest, so hopefully that will help out with the arms.

I told my sister that I don't remember chemo being this hard - I was lucky with chemo. It can be very hard on some people, but Linda did state that I had some hard chemo days. I just don't remember; must be the chemo brain.
I am running out of space and so I will let you go. Thanks again for all your support-

Here's to a sunny day soon!
LOL

Posted Feb 20, 2008 4:45pm

I keep forgetting to tell you that I have hair, eye brows, and eye lashes again!!!!! In fact, my eye brows are bushy and I am thinking of waxing them to have them nicely shaped. As many of you know, fashion was not my forte - jeans, sweatshirt, and gym shoes is what I am most comfortable in - but when I lost my hair and didn't feel very lady-like (as I did in my jeans and sweatshirt) I actually started to dress (most of the time) like a woman on my days off; something that I never really did before. (I would dress up for when I subbed last year but never on a day off.) I would even make sure that I had on more jewelry then normal. But with the return of my hair, I may go back to my comfortable days - we shall see.

There is a group of women in Kenosha that meet once a month (informally) and I might start going to their meetings. It is on Thursday nights and Becca has gymnastics until 9:00pm so this could work out really well since I stay up anyways for Becca. I will let you know how it goes, but I am hoping that it is what I have been looking for since September.

My car won't be ready until tomorrow afternoon - and that is about it for the day. We are supposed to get a heat wave this weekend. Do enjoy the slush.

See ya' later

Posted Feb 27, 2008 5:13pm

OK-I had written something yesterday but hit a wrong button – AGAIN - and lost what I had typed. So what does a 40 yr-old mature woman do when that happens? She walks away from the computer and curses it.

I am not sure how many radiation treatments I have done but I have 3/31 as my last day on my mind. I think that I will be done then as long as the machine doesn't go down.

Today at treatment as I was putting on my beautiful pink robe when I noticed an outline of the cross that I wear on my skin. I suppose if I am to be branded with something that a cross is pretty high up on the list. Now my necklace is not tight and I don't wear tight shirts (not being contoured, I can't show off the ladies that well, yet) so I am not sure why the marks. I just am not going to wear the cross until the radiation treatments end. I can't remember the last time I didn't wear a cross on a regular basis - but I am sure God will understand.

The treatments are getting much faster. I think I was only there for about 10 minutes today. I found the shortest way to Lake Forest from Kenosha. I was able to cut out about 336 miles over the 28 days - almost a tank of gas (on a cheap day) so that is helpful. And I am listening to *An Old Man and a Fish* by Ernest Hemingway. I am really enjoying the book. My car is in the shop today so I don't know the end of the book yet, but hopefully by the end of the week I will have the story done.

My arms (mostly the left) are still a bit sore and I don't have full range yet; I am hoping soon, but I am not sure how long this will take. I do my exercises daily and tomorrow I have physical therapy. I will go to physical therapy 8 times over a 4 week period. I find it much easier to work with someone then

89

by myself, and that is why my walking buddies really helped me. When this ice is gone, I will be calling upon the ladies again to strut our stuff!!! (And there will be no bouncing for me!!!)

Rob and I went out Saturday for a fund raiser for a local school. It was Vegas style with 21 tables. I gambled and won some raffle tickets. With the tickets you dropped them in a container, hoping to win whatever the item is.

Sidetrack here - what am I going to do after chemo, surgery and radiation? I am going to Disney World, of course!

Back to the night out - there was a container for 4 one day hopper passes for Disney and yes I won the big item of the evening!!! I almost went home early too. I was tired, but it was nice to be out and about and seeing people that I haven't seen most of the winter.

I am so excited about the sunshine and the warm days that seem to be coming more and more frequently, even though I know that there will be a few more days of winter.
I need to finish cooking and getting dinner ready. Not only does radiation take up a lot of time, but so does getting back to doing some of the things that I haven't done on a consistent basis.

Talk to you later
Thanks again for the support
And here's to SPRING! I believe and have faith that it will be here soon.

Love to all

Posted Mar 3, 2008 5:30pm

I received the letter today officially letting me know that I didn't win the bedroom make-over (and yes I am a bit bummed because I had rearranged my house to accommodate the new room). Thank you for your support. They received over 1500 entries. I would say better luck next year but I am not doing this again. Once in my life is enough.

I was asked by a couple of people about staying so positive, but I will let you know that not every day is a happy one for me. I definitely have hard days with this journey that was thrust upon me, but I really do try to keep the gloom and doom thoughts and feelings to a minimum - otherwise I probably would put my head in the sand (if I can get through the ice and snow that is).

I will have to write later - no one seems to be able to be alone at the moment!
Talk to you soon

Posted Mar 6, 2008 10:10pm

Hello again.
Well my radiation seems to be going OK. The skin feels tighter but the feeling doesn't last all day. I went to another PT appt. That is a godsend. It is really helping me get the motion back in my arms.

Did I tell you not only do I get hot flashes but I think that I am getting cold flashes as well? I am sitting in my house with my coat on as I type on the computer and I am freezing. It drives me nuts that my body cannot regulate its temperature to one zone.

I met a woman who has breast cancer (last year was her journey) and she invited me to meet with other women who have breast cancer and they are closer to my age; the oldest is 51. Some have kids that are a bit younger than Raney and Becca. Tonight was the first meeting for me. I think that these women have been meeting for about 3-4 years. I am hoping that this will work out for me because it would be nice to hear if they lose it and yell at their children for no reason and that I am not crazy and that I will get through this and my kids will survive me. I think that there were about 8 women in the group.

I should probably reread the side effects of the tamoxifen. I can't seem to get my head on straight today - more so than my new normal lack of brain. I am bouncing all around today.

But today was a good day. It was so sunny and I love that. I could have used a few more degrees, but sun is a good starting point. I went shopping for the girls today. I am not ready to shop for me because I am not finished being contoured yet - but watch out when it is all said and done! With the non-sagging breasts who knows what types of shirts I might venture to wear.

I am getting tired but I don't know if that is from the radiation or because I am staying up later now that I feel better. (Not perfect yet but way better!!!!) I will be really thrilled when I can sleep on my side and there is no pain. At least I can sneeze and it doesn't hurt me anymore.

I thought that there was something that I wanted to share but I tell you this: brain-fried.

We have had a pretty good week with getting homework done and the kids to bed a bit earlier than normal. That helps with the morning being smoother. I hope everyone is doing well. I am going to go to bed and Raney is in her own bed at the moment so we shall see how the night goes. Perhaps tonight I will be able to sleep through the night.

Talk to you later

Posted Mar 8, 2008 7:15pm

Good Evening - the last of the nights before the time change. I am so excited about gaining more light. Now on to heat; and I am not talking hot flashes.

I still have no brain because I had thought about something to share and now I can't even remember the topic. Hopefully it will come back to me because I am sure it was full of wisdom and could change your life.

I took over Rob's gym membership and I am starting back on the treadmill. I am not sure when the snow and ice will melt enough for the walkers of Kenosha to get back out, but I know we will all be looking forward to walking outside again. I walked only about 2.5 miles today. It is not as much fun as outside and with friends. Support is a wonderful way to keep me motivated.

Today we had a pizza party for some family birthdays and then we went to the Brat Stop in Kenosha. They were having a fundraiser for St. Baldrick's cancer fund for childhood cancers. People raised money and then had their hair shaved off. I think people thought I shaved my head. I did see one woman have her head shaved. I heard that last year seven women shaved their heads. They are hoping to raise $100,000. Raney wanted to have her head shaved so I told her next year; one baldy at a time in my house. I don't want anyone fighting with me over hats and bandanas. It was a nice time though, lots of silent auction items.

I wish I could remember things. Maybe someday, but I am not hopeful. Rob and I are going to help celebrate a 50th birthday tonight for a neighbor. I love birthday parties and I am going to two today.

My skin is not too red. They said that it might start to look like **a really bad sunburn**. I think I've had 12 treatments and so far the skin is hanging tough. I am hoping for that the whole time so I can shock the doctors again.

I better get going. I can't remember the last time that I went out at this time of the evening; lately this is almost my bedtime. I am able to stay up later now. I have most of my energy back, but my arm does get tired much quicker than before.

Good night and sweet dreams--
Love to ya!

Posted Mar 11, 2008 6:35pm

Good Evening everyone-
I am not sure what number of zapping I am on but the skin is still looking OK and my x-rays (yes I get x-rayed once a week; I am not getting enough through radiation so they find ways to zap me more) are looking good. I looked at them once when they were showing me where they are zapping me. My expanders are part of the picture; very strange looking.

I was counting one day the number of men that have seen me topless since

93

August. I think it was around 9 and then on Monday at radiation - where it has been all female therapists - there was another man. Not that I am even fazed anymore. I just think of strange things sometimes in the car.

I might start taking the train down and riding my bike to the hospital; it would only be about a 2-3 mile bike ride, but talk about being green. And what better month to start then St. Paddy's month (Becca has been wearing green everyday to school since March 1st - Raney won't - something about the sprites will get mad).

I am having another hot flash; these suck! I watch my neck and face get red in the mirror. Better than the TV shows that are on these days.
My energy level is OK. I have heard that radiation can wipe you out, and I read about that in a book, but so far not too bad. I am still able to get the girls to bed. And then I try to read for a bit or I just go to bed at the same time. My arm sometimes gets tired so then I stop doing whatever it is that I am doing. It's hard sometimes with these new limits because I tried to do most of the stuff around the house, but I am getting better at asking for help.

I just wish I would get my brain back.

Now I remember the story I wanted to share. Becca and I were talking about shampoo and somehow I told her that I wash my hair. She thought that was very funny. I guess to an 8 yr-old short hair doesn't need shampoo. I didn't tell her about the conditioning.

I can put my right arm straight up into the air next to my ear; my left arm still needs some work, but it is getting so much better. Just a couple of months ago I couldn't put on my coat by myself and now I am back to wearing over-the-head shirts and sweaters.

I almost have a month's worth of tamoxifen done. That means 29-59 months left to go. Doesn't that seem like a long time? I am hoping that it doesn't cause hot flashes the whole time.

Have a great night...sweet dreams

Happy St Paddy's Day!

I am not sure what my week was like last week so therefore it must have been uneventful - thank God!!!!

This weekend I took Becca to the Irish Heritage Center so that she can get in touch with her Irish side. It was a nice time. Rob made corn beef yesterday and some of the family came over to enjoy the meal, but not me or Becca!!!

My skin is starting to show the effects of radiation and I am tired, but I don't know if that is from radiation or just my children not letting me sleep. There are certain areas that are getting sore on the left side as well but nothing too major. I have to remember after radiation that I am doing something that my body doesn't like.

I had therapy for my arms today and I am doing very well in that area. I can move my left arm 130 degrees; I feel it but it isn't too bad. Soon it will be back to what it was.

Rob, Raney, Becca, and I are going to MO for Easter and then Rob and I are coming home Monday without the kids. They are going to hang out with Aunt Diane and Uncle Howard for spring break. I will be going to radiation over spring break, but at least I won't be getting Raney and Becca up and out for that week. Then I will only have one more treatment left!!!! The countdown has begun, 9 left to go!!!!!!

I need to pick up the rug rats from school and see how their day went.

May the luck of the Irish be with you!!!
LOL

Happy Spring, or so the calendar states.
I have three radiations left on my neck area and 6 left on the chest area!!!
According to Dr. Imperato my skin is looking good and I am doing well. My
skin is bothering me a little in the back but nothing to really write home
about. I think that it could be a whole lot worse.

We leave at the crack of dawn tomorrow to get to MO (radiation first) and
then spring break for the kiddies.

My arm therapist is amazed at my energy level. (She doesn't see me at
9:00pm.) I too thought my energy would be way down from what I read, but
so far it isn't that bad. And my arm really moves now, not 100% but close. I
will be ready for the summer.

I know this is choppy and going to be short, but I need to get a few things
done before I head off to get the girls.

Happy Easter!!!!

Well I am done being zapped in the neck area and only three more to go in
the chest area!!!! I found out today that I have breast tissue left so
therefore I am not 100% fake!! I didn't know that.

Easter was nice. We left Kenosha before the big snow storm and when we
got to Columbia it was in the high 60's!!! It felt like FL. Rob even went
golfing. Becca, Raney, and I went to a park across the street every day. It
was just nice to get outside with no winter coat.

Monday morning, Rob and I left the girls in MO. They are having a great
vacation and I don't have to drag them to my zapping sessions. It is a win-
win for all involved. I am not sure if the girls are going to want to come

home. They don't sound homesick (which is a very good thing seeing they are about 8 hrs from us).

The house is so quiet, but Rob and I are taking advantage of the kid less time: we went out to dinner and maybe tonight we will go somewhere for a drink. Thursday we are going out to dinner with some friends.

Other than that, nothing else is really going on. I am not sure if after radiation I follow up with this dr. or if I go my merry way. I need to try and remember to ask him.

My hair looks to me like a two-yr-old boy who just got his hair cut for the summer! But today I went and had my eyebrows waxed and shaped. A girly thing to do because I keep telling Rob that I am not playboy material anymore (not that I really ever was but now I am really off the charts), so it was nice to do something that probably only women do.

I better get going and enjoy the peace and quiet of the house.
Until we chat again
Have a wonderful day

Love to all

Posted Mar 30, 2008 4:37pm

Rob and I stayed at my cousin's on Friday night and we picked up the girls Saturday. I received a few calls asking me if I actually went and got the girls. It was a quiet week without them and as nice as it was, I am glad that I am back with my girls. Rob worked out of the house all week, but it still was a little too quiet for my liking.

I have only 1 zap session left!!!!!!!!

After this, I visit with Dr. Imperato in 6 weeks and then I take him out of my fab five - I don't need to follow up with him after that. He is happy with the way my skin looks; it bothers me a little bit, but I have seen worse. My throat has been sore on and off these 28 days, but I am not sure that it is from radiation or something in the air.

I am currently on my own for arm therapy. I was told that if I don't stay on top of the 25 exercises they gave me, I might end up needing rotor cuff surgery. I have seen that up close so I will be very good about stretching and working the arms.

After tomorrow, I only have follow ups with 3 doctors.

I am now on what is referred to as "The Leap of Faith". There are no scans to look again inside my bones and organs. I just need to r...lost my thought...I just need to believe that everything was done perfectly. It is hard to do that; I want a piece of paper promising me old age, but I will learn to embrace Faith so please keep the prayers coming (and add some to help me have the strength and courage to believe all is right within my body).

I need to think about dinner and what we are going to do on our last spring break night...
Have a wonderful night and week

Talk to you soon

Posted Mar 31, 2008 8:55pm

Good Evening
Well it's official: I have leapt off the cliff and am riding on that wave of faith; so far it's good. I was given a certificate of punctuality, corporation and positive attitude; I got the gold star. I'm a good cancer patient. I did what they told me and, to this day, I still never really felt like a patient (except for the surgery part - that hurt the most and made the most physical change - there is no hiding that one).

What does one do to celebrate the end of all treatments?? Cold Stone Creamery! I was told I needed to celebrate and I am always willing to celebrate something. It was a better idea than letting the ladies run free around the block "It's over and I still don't bounce" (that would be topless, for those that are not thinking along with my bad sense of humor).

I have no doctor appointments for the month of April - Who knows what I can accomplish with all this time back! Speaking of time, I am gathering the troops again for walking. I don't think spring is coming but at least it is not bitter cold, so I have my walking shoes ready and waiting by the front door.

The rest of my words of wisdom will have to wait since Raney is not going to sleep as well as she should, and to have a better morning I better go see what she needs.

THANK YOU FOR YOUR SUPPORT AND LOVE through this process--but please keep the prayers coming--I NEVER!!! want to do this again. As many good things that have come my way over these eight months, I don't need to re-run this journey.

LOVE TO ALL

Posted Apr 5, 2008 8:39am

I need to update the pictures so you can see me with my new locks of hair! Actually my hair has never been flatter and it looks like the plastic hair on dolls, but hey, it's hair!!!

I met with my support group again. They were being interviewed for a magazine called *She*. It is a free publication for this area. I am not sure if it is going to go into IL. The writer was going to write an article about the group and if people wanted to join - that kind of thing.

It's funny (not ha-ha funny) but as we were chatting about our new lives a lady shared how her husband didn't want her doing a living will. Rob didn't even want to discuss it with me, but I kept badgering him. No papers were drawn up, but I made it perfectly clear what my wishes were. It helped me knowing that I wasn't the only one who thought these thoughts, and that Rob wasn't the only one who had a hard time with the idea. To me it is a no-brainer, but then I wasn't on the side of making really difficult decision if things went that way.

Everyone in the group felt that getting this journey was not something to choose but because we are on it we see it is full of amazing gifts. I have all of you to thank for that. I am still awed by all the support and prayers (and I still need them, so don't go away). I will tell you what is next on my list; it is quite the need - almost ranks with staying on this planet! It is nice to be with people who have been to hell and back and have a smile on their face, hair on their heads, and they tell it like it is. No sugar coating here. Life stays good - even with cancer.

There is a woman (she had a double mastectomy) and she stated last time that she hates her breasts. I have been wondering about this for awhile because I don't like mine either. I am glad I have some, but they don't look or feel good; they are just weird. In this group I can ask anything, so I asked about what she didn't like about them and her statements could have been mine. I was hoping that I might like them someday and maybe I will, but at least I am not alone in my thoughts. I don't like changing in the locker room when I work out. I didn't think about changing shirts until I was already there. I was panicked that someone might see me and scream in horror. I realize that this is irrational and no one would do that, but I am not the most rational grape in the bunch.

Back to the breasts. This woman got her nipples 3 months ago and she showed them. They look real, but she informed me that not all nipples will take and that is where you all need to pray for me. When I am there (and it will be a long time) I will need prayers to save the nipples. (Wouldn't that be an interesting T-shirt to wear??) I will let you know when it's time for that one. See how fun this can get???? Just for the record though, this woman is happy and not bitter. She, like me, just wanted to keep the real ones. I even told the ladies that I forgot what they felt like. So here is my plug for you ladies reading today.

FEEL YOURSELF MONTHLY!!!!! If this was something that I had done, maybe the outcome of the surgery would have been different - and if not, it would have been an easier recovery (my right side is in much better shape than the left side) and my lymph nodes would have survived. And breast cancer doesn't run in the family which seems to be the case with a lot of the women in my support group. Ladies, check your breasts!!!! I am off the soap box now.

And my wise words for the day:
Cancer can take a physical life, but it cannot stop me from having a life!!!!!! I am living through this all!!~!~~. Thanks for the prayers. I would not have made it without you.

Love and lots of it to all

Good morning everyone! We are having another glorious spring day in Kenosha. It's breezy, 70 degrees, and sunny!!! So I took my leap of faith, and I must not have read the manual because I crashed into the first brick wall.

Monday April 7th: I got up, got the kids to school, and went grocery shopping (I used totes - trying to eliminate plastic bags from my house), did a little laundry; I was having a NORMAL day. Rob grilled out for dinner and then we went for a walk in the park (sounds nice huh?).

Before our walk was done, I needed to get home because I started to feel very uncomfortable. My left side - where I was zapped for 28 days was really starting to bother me. I went to bed at 8:15pm. By the morning it hurt as bad as surgery to get in and out of bed. God and I will have a chat about my language that night because the bladder still wanted to do its job. I spent most of the evening awake. I also got the chills a few times that evening. One time a hot flash and the chills joined forces to torture me - in case you are wondering, the chills won. Who would have thought that??

Tues 4/8: Rob and I went to see Dr. Imperato and he thought that I had a skin infection called cellulitis. He put me on antibiotics. My left side was warm to the touch and looked swollen. And did I mention Hurts like HELL!!!! When Rob and I got home, I went upstairs and didn't come down until Wed.

Wed 4/9: Rob and I went downtown to see the plastic surgeon. He was not my doctor but a partner, so they had me return on Thur. I went to bed around 7:45pm.

Thurs 4/10: Dr. Fine wasn't sure that it was an infection; he thought it might be a reaction to the radiation. He told me to stay on the antibiotics - just in case it was an infection - and to come back in two weeks. He also said that it might be that my body and implants are not going to work, which means I would need to use tissue in the future if I want to keep breasts. I am really hoping that I don't have to go that route. Surgery and recovery is longer. So I am in a 'wait and see' mode. But at least the pain is less and I stayed up until 8:00pm. I had a hard time falling asleep, but at least I was lying down.

Fri: No doctor visits and I stayed awake until 9:30pm. The pain is a lot less - it is still tender but nothing like before. God loves me still, even with the potty mouth.

I need to give credit to Rob; he was quite the nurse. He made sure that I took my meds and asked me if I needed anything throughout the day. The highest temperature that I am aware I had was 101.6, but I am now fever free. I had asked Dr. Fine when I could call and cry like a baby and he said if the fever was over 101 or the breasts changed. I am still sore, but nothing like last Monday, and no fever so something is going in the right direction.

I hope you all had a much better week than me - again this isn't pain that I would wish on my worst enemy. My spark is back and I'm ready to fight the good fight again (good fight, is there such a thing?).

Tonight my new cancer support group is meeting with the husbands - 1st time in 3 yrs - and I am not sure that we are going to go. I think that the tiredness of getting zapped has found me and then the pain of whatever it was last week has really taken me down a few notches. I really wanted to go because I think that Rob really would have benefitted being with males that are in the same boat as he is.

Remember
I AM WOMAN HEAR ME ROAR!!!

Nothing is going to keep me down for long. I have many people that are cheering me on. And remember, this is the month of our big walk. April 27th - if you want to join us to walk, email me and let me know.

Thanks again for all your love and support. I couldn't do this VERY bumpy journey without you.

Lots of love (or lol as Raney will say)

Hello Friends,
I am tired today. I took the kids to a Girl Scout camp in East Troy, WI for Laura Ingalls Day. They showed us how big the covered wagon was, the cabin, how they made cornmeal, braided rugs, and other things. It was really interesting. I am not sure how I would do in the 1800s. I might have to read some of her books, which she didn't start writing until she was 65 yrs old. What an amazing life story. I told Rob today that my life story is not that amazing yet, so I better get going.

I think Raney and Becca are happy with me. Raney was talking about something that I used to do when they didn't weigh too much and I pretended that they were in a washing machine. I would then pick them up to hang them to dry. That was nice to listen to. Sometimes I wonder what my children remember.
I better go; I thought the girls were watching a movie and that doesn't seem to be the case.

I will write more later.

This is the second time I've tried to type out my 100th update. You would think by 100 that I would know how to do an update but for some reason I don't – another story.

I went and saw Dr. Fine last Thursday and interestingly, at least to him, is that they are not reacting to the antibiotics the way he expected. I am not sure that I want me or even my body parts to be interesting to a Dr. - now if I was dating him that might be another story...but who really wants to be an interesting patient???? I want to be BORING!!!!!

I get to see Dr. Fine again this Thursday. Hopefully, I bore him and he doesn't want to see me for months! Trust me, my heart will not be broken. (He is a very nice doctor and very kind, but this weekly relationship can end.)

Yesterday was our big walk - Raney hit about 76% of her goal!
THANK YOU for all your support.

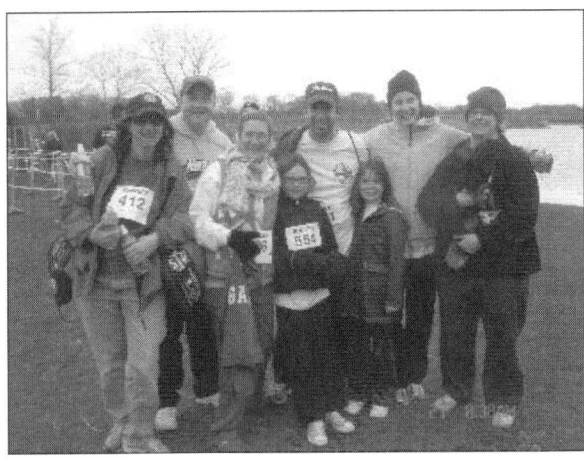

Here is the group: Eileen, Rob, Jimee, Kristin, Katy, Valentine, Becca and Raney - we also had lots of "in spirit walkers"!!!

I posted pictures from that and Easter. Check out the new do. (My 2 yr-old boy hair cut.) Jimee tells me that I have hair like my mom, salt and pepper, but I think that I am pepper and salt. An 8th grader at the school told me that I look like a young Jamie Lee Curtis. I told her that I was going to take her home and she could compliment me daily! She told me she charges $10 an hour.

Eileen, Jimee, Kristin, Katy, and Valentine joined Rob, Raney, Becca and me for the 5k. Jimee and Becca finished in about 34 minutes; Rob, Kristin, and Raney finished in about 44 minutes.

Katy, Eileen, Valentine and I finished in about 1 hr and 9 minutes - we were so not about rushing. We would have stopped and smelled the flowers but due to the cold weather there were no flowers to smell.

It is a beautiful place to walk - Independence Grove in Libertyville, IL if you ever get a chance to go out there.
We started our day at 5:30am. I needed to make sure that I had time for my tea without having the kids awake. I need time to wake up - mornings last a long time when you wake up that early - but my evening was cut very short. By 7:30pm I went to bed. I have finally figured out how to get my 9 yr-old in her own bed: go to bed before her. Who would have known that is the secret???

I am still sore in the radiated area but that is normal. I don't think I am as red as I was before so I do think that I am on the road to recovery. I will really be quite the happy camper when the pain goes away - those chest muscles are involved in almost every movement I make. I guess I didn't appreciate my body enough when I had it good, so when I am back to being me my body is going to be treated like the gift that it is.

I need to feed the munchkins and send them to bed. My lack of energy and their high level sometimes really don't mix – we can be like oil and water.

I still believe that spring is going to make it to the Midwest; I just hope it happens before we are to have winter again.

Happy day to all

I am not sure what I am doing wrong; you would think that after all this time I would have this down to a science, but maybe I still have chemo brain, who knows.

I wrote something of great importance yesterday and now I can't remember much of it. I do know that I was sharing with my lady friends that there are no more mammograms for me (only 1.5 in this lifetime), but you all need to go get those boobs smashed!!!! Don't put it off - 1 out 8 women will be diagnosed and the number of women where it is not in the family is on the rise. (OK, no more lecturing on that in this update, but just please know it is a VERY important thing to do. I wouldn't wish this journey on my worst enemy.)

I saw the plastic surgeon, Dr Fine, today. He just cracks me up. I don't think he has ever yelled in his life, he is so soft-spoken, and I still remain 'interesting' to him. The last time I saw him he told me we were going to wait longer to replace the implants with the permanent ones; today he said we are moving forward with the swap on June 29th. My skin looks unhappy - how happy is it supposed to be when it got cut open, parts removed, and then radiated for 28 days?? He said that I have some purple spots that he doesn't like and that my skin is thin; so no more expanding for me. I never even got the chance to decide if I wanted to be bigger. So 2 cups sizes smaller than before surgery is where I will stay. The surgery is day surgery and should only take an hour and half.

I saw the oncologist last week; she has me on a shot, Zoladex, which I thought I was getting once and then I was done with it. I don't ask the right questions! This shot is every three months for the next 5 years. I need a book that tells me "what questions to ask your doctor". I am hoping to be able to do this shot locally. I like Chicago, but I don't want to have to go downtown every three months for one shot.

One more thing and then off to bed.

My sister-in-law, Sole, was diagnosed with breast cancer 5 years ago and then again about the same time I was. She has a very aggressive cancer that has moved to her organs. I would like you to send her and her girls prayers that they may get the guidance that they need at this time in their lives. I know that the 3-day walk and Avon's walks are coming up with the "nice" weather that we are having. If you are donating, please add an extra dollar, so that a cure can be found so that my nieces and all future females/males, who could be on this potential path have a better fighting chance - or no need to be on it at all!!!!!.
We all deserve a lifetime.

Thanks so much

P.S. one great thing this cancer has brought me is coming up this weekend: I am going to hang out with some of my college friends; some of them I haven't seen in years. We decided it was time to get together. Cancer can really make you stop and smell the roses.

Posted Jun 2, 2008 7:31pm

Being raised with 5 brothers, 3 sisters, and many visiting cousins, one learns to be flexible. So I went with the flow when Dr. Fine's office called today and said that there was an opening for surgery this Friday. So I am going this Friday to have the temporaries removed and the "permanent" (someone told me they last 12 years) ones put in. I am hoping that this will take away some of the pain that I have; but there goes my chances of being a triple D.

My college weekend was a lot fun but as they say, "what happens in Vegas stays in Vegas"; so what happens in Oak Park stays in Oak Park (right ladies!!) I am just kidding. We were well behaved and had a lot of fun catching up.

I need to go and hang out with Raney and Becca, so good night all.

This is going to be a quickie - just like surgery today (only 2 hours). I was put under with twilight sedation. I just stressed VERY heavily that I didn't want to feel anything or remember anything (too many horror movies in my past). I came out unscathed.

Rob and I left at 5:30am; way too early, especially since I wasn't able to have my tea!!! But once we got there I was taken in the back pretty quickly. I was not in the Prentice Hospital for women, so my room did not have a plasma TV (bummer). I was much calmer and probably would have watched something to help pass a little time. Believe it or not, I am quiet when I get up at 5:30am.

I don't remember being taken away or brought back. I was sent home after about an hour in recovery.

I will share a few stories early next week, for now I am going to bed.

Good Night and sleep tight

Sole, my sister-in-law
Posted Aug 15, 2008 5:05pm

Hi
I am doing well and I now have bed-head again. In fact I even have had a haircut already.

As many of you know, my sister-in-law, Sole, was diagnosed for a 2nd time around the same time that I was last year; this time for a very aggressive cancer. Sole (and her family) are dealing with the very ugly cancer. Sole fought as long as she could and took any option the doctor talked to her about; she was always saying, yes, yes let's keep on trying. I read somewhere that cancer cannot kill the spirit and that is so true in Sole's case. Sole is a woman of strength and courage beyond measure.

We are being told by hospice that she might have a week because of her spirit, but she is in a coma and there is no response. Sole is coming home tonight to be surrounded by her family (her sister is here from Bolivia) and God's love. This is the start of the end of the journey for Sole. Please pray for peace and guidance for Sole to join Kevin (my brother, her husband) and the rest of her family in heaven. I know that Sole is so sad leaving Earth, but will rejoice in reuniting with her family on the other side.

I am going to go on my soap box ladies: look into the eyes of your loved ones and promise them that you will get a mammogram before the end of the year. Most new breast cancer cases have no family history which means YOU need to get the boobies smashed for a few uncomfortable minutes to help keep you healthy!!!! Early detection is key in the battle against breast cancer.

Again if you have the opportunity to help out with breast cancer research by buying stamps, Campbell's tomato soup, or whatever else is out there, please consider doing it so that the Soles of the world no longer have to go through this journey.

We all deserve a lifetime.
Thanks and LOL to all of you

Sole's announcement
Posted Aug 19, 2008 10:50am

Thanks again for all your prayers. Again, Sole battled breast cancer twice - please pray for a cure so that no one else has to endure the ugliness of this cancer.

Soledad Dunn, 50, of St. Charles. Sole was the loving wife of the late Kevin Dunn, and mother of Cecila, Angi and Andrea; Sister of Lucila, Ana, Patrico and Wilfredo; daughter of the late Angela Zeballos and Santiago Barba. . Born July 24, 1958, in Santa Cruz, Boliva. Sole was an expert seamstress and an even better mother. Full of life and love, Sole was a joy to friends and family. Her smile and laughter will be remembered by all who knew her. Visitation will be from 4 p.m. to 9 p.m., Thursday, August 21 at Williams-

Kampp Funeral Home, 430 E. Roosevelt Rd. (1 block E. of Naperville Rd.) Wheaton. Funeral Friday, August 22, 9:15 a.m. to St. Patrick's Church, 6N491 Crane Road, St. Charles, IL, Mass 10:30 a.m. Interment St. Mary Cemetery, Fremont Center, IL.

Sole was 50 years old.

Posted Sep 13, 2008 3:14am

Hi--I know that it has been awhile since I have written. I was living my life: taking the kids to the beach, walks, and whatever summer seemed to want us to do, and of course the beginning of school and feeling good. I am ready for a better year.

We went to my brother-in-law's summer home in Northern WI. This summer I ended up sleeping on the couch and I woke up with a very sore back. I went to a chiropractor to see if that would help and it didn't really. When I saw the oncologist (this appointment was after Sole had died) I told her that I was full of complaints because I was scared. I know a couple of women who had the breast cancer spread to their spines. The doctor ordered a MRI that I did on Sept 4. The results came back with suspicious spots on my spine. Little did I know that would have been wonderful if that was all it was. Then a bone and cat scan were ordered. I did those tests on the 10th. I now have the knowledge of spots on my liver, lung and spine. A biopsy has been scheduled for Monday morning on the liver - the day after my 41st birthday. I can't seem to get a good birthday in so I think that I might skip the 40's and move straight to the very young 50's.

The reason the liver is chosen is because it is the easiest to get to and the results are in faster - and I am all about fast in this area of my life.
I did ask if this could be something else and the PA (physician assistant) said yes, but she really didn't think so. She said that it looks like the breast cancer has spread, but that it is still very treatable. I will know more on Wednesday after meeting with the doctor to talk about results. My brother Jimee will be joining Rob and I for that meeting because he was so well behaved at all the other meetings last year; it's really because even though Rob and I listen, Jimee hears the important things.

110

Yes, I am completely freaked out about this and I have already been telling Rob what kind of stepmom I want for my kids (I don't think Rob found my wicked sense of humor funny). My mom would have thought that was funny.

My test is at 9:30am Monday. If you remember, please send a quick prayer that would be great.

I worked today as the gym teacher and tomorrow is the Kindergarten Room!!!

I certainly didn't hear what I wanted to (and I am still waiting for some results) but this is the quick version: I have breast cancer that has spread to my spine in three different areas, my liver, and tiny spots on my lung. This makes my cancer Stage 4.

I will be starting chemo again next Friday; another chance for those who weren't able to make it to come join in the fun of watching me get chemo! We hang out, talk, make cards, etc. I will have chemo two Fridays in a row and then one week off. I am going to do this for two months and then I will be re-scanned and we will assess the situation at that time to see what the next step will be. My understanding is I will be on something for the rest of my life to manage the cancer - there is only remission for me, no more cure - but as I told the PA I can live with remission; it's the other road that I can't live with.

I am getting a new port on Friday. Because I was so sure that I was never going to need it again, I had it removed in Jan.

For the medical audience, I will be on Gemzer, Zometa, and Avastin. I don't get all three every time, but I don't remember the cycles - Jimee wrote that down for me.

I did have a day of believing this was the end and that I wasn't going to be here to watch Raney and Becca graduate grammar school, but that day is

111

over and I am now just getting ready to being the best manager of my body possible.

The other good news - and then I will have to let you go because I am off to a band meeting – is that Raney is going to learn the clarinet this year!! And, my spleen, adrenals, pancreas, bile ducts and kidneys are normal. Every bit helps!!!
But the spine and liver are not so lucky (they use the word extensive) but remember, I respond well to medicine, so I just need to do it again.

Thanks so much and I will chat with you later

Hello Everyone-

Rob is getting rid of grass clippings and getting a hamster with the girls - so I have a few minutes of peace and quiet.

I am not sure if I wrote the results from the liver biopsy. It came back positive for cancer, so they are making the assumption that it is also in the spine and lung.
I am ER+, so that is a good thing, and PR - I am not sure what would be different if it's positive and I am still waiting on the hur2 test. If positive, it just offers different options.

What I get to do this week to get ready for my new life: on Friday I have yet another blood draw; on Monday (I am going to have low blood counts because everyone keeps taking it - and they also throw some of it away (not a nice thing to do since I just got stuck!!!) I get to fill up about 3-5 tubes; Wednesday I get my brain scanned (I am doing this test in Kenosha) to see if I have anything upstairs - it has been questionable lately, but the real reason is to make sure I don't have cancer in the brain because that would make a change in the game plan; Thursday night Rob and I are going to stay at my brother's friend's place in Evanston to be downtown by 7 am for a new and improved port, chemo's best friend. Then I will go upstairs to the floor with a beautiful view and get chemo - again. Two weeks on, one week off. I do this for a couple of months and then re-scan to see if it's working.

My sister bought a book about eating differently to help stop cancer cell growth so I am now trying new foods and they are really good, even dark chocolate is on the list. (Red wine is also on the list, but I am not sure I will be taking advantage of that because of the liver.) Black tea is off the list, but I am drinking green tea. But otherwise it doesn't seem too hard to follow.

Raney and I imagine Pac-man eating my cancer cells then Pac-man leaves the body, throwing the cancer cells away and going to another person with cancer. Then we fill up my areas (and the other people with cancer) with God's healing light, say a couple of prayers and go to sleep. Becca will be joining us when I catch her at a good time to explain this to her. I tried last night but we both were too tired.

I am going to back track here. Back to the Monday of the liver biopsy: they had to use a larger needle then I usually have (small veins) and the reason was in case I bleed out - which of course freaks me out - I didn't think about anything going wrong and my dark side came out as I told Rob, "Well, good luck. Linda can help you with the bills and be nice to Raney and Becca." Rob did not think that was funny, but I made my mom laugh up in heaven because that is something that she would have said. As you know, everything went fine and I am still someone who has a dark sense of humor.

Thanks for the prayers and thoughts. I know that I will have many more days that are harder to be positive than before but I will manage this disease to the best of my ability and take one day at a time. All the support that I get will keep me going strong.

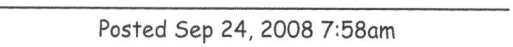

Posted Sep 24, 2008 7:58am

Hello
I forgot to send this out yesterday to get my troops ready, so please forgive me. Today is the day that my brain gets scanned, and, of course, I woke up with a headache (I don't get these too often). So of course, I have a brain

tumor, and I will be rushed immediately into surgery - wouldn't that explain my lack of memory!! I am so KIDDING!!!!

I really don't think anything is going to go wrong, but it never hurts to have a few prayers - say around 9:30am! Thanks so much to everyone for all the love and support that Rob, the girls, and I have been getting. It really helps beyond any measure.

I subbed yesterday and I am taking the rest of the week off. I have a spa day and I need to make sure that the house is in order for me to come home nice and relaxed.

I will have to let you go so I can look pretty for the pictures, but I have lots of thoughts to share with you.

Mentally, I am doing a whole lot better. I can walk into Raney and Becca's room while they are sleeping (on that rare occasion that someone isn't sleeping next to me) and not cry; I even smile now. See I am at the top of the world and am ready to FACE the giant to win!!!!!!!!

Have a wonderful day and do something soon that is special that you have put on your back burner: break out the china, get a massage, walk to the lake, see a movie, etc. We all have some living to do!!!!

See you later

Round II
Posted Sep 26, 2008 5:32pm

Patty has just finished round II and is on her way home. The port was put in this morning, finishing up around 10:45am. Patty was sore, but there were no complications. The Chemo treatment didn't start until about 2:00pm and Patty finished about 4:30pm.

This was to be the longest chemo day.
The first phase of round II:

Patty has chemo two weeks on and one week off for 3 weeks.
Then she gets scanned again.
DATE # DRUGS APPROXIMATE TIME FOR EACH DRUG
9/26 3 drugs - 90 minutes; 30-60 minutes; 15 minutes
10/3 1 drug - 30 to 60 minutes
10/10 OFF YEAH.
10/17 2 drugs - 60 minutes; 30 - 60 minutes
10/24 2 drugs - 30-60 minutes; 15 minutes
10/31 OFF - CELEBRATE HALLOWEEN
11/7 2 drugs - 30 minutes; 30-60 minutes
11/14 1 drug - 30-60 minutes
11/21 OFF
Re-scanned

Hope you all are doing well.
Jimee

Posted Sep 29, 2008 8:31am

Good Morning
I love my children so much. They bought me a shell vase with a beautiful
rose. They bought me this rose/shell vase because I fainted 2 times on Sat.
First at 5:00 a.m. then at 9:30 a.m.

To back up a bit, Friday after chemo we went home with very little traffic
and I made myself some dinner. I was feeling quite OK. I did take a pain pill
because the port spot hurt but I slept like a baby until around 5:00am when
I needed to go to the bathroom. When I got up, I was dizzy, so I lay down
but then I felt like I was going to throw up so I had to get up. On my way
back to bed I must have passed out because Rob was by my side asking me
what happened. How am I supposed to know? He watched me for about a half
hour (and this is a pet peeve of mine -to be stared at) before he believed
that I was going to continue to breath and be OK.

Then 9:30am rolled around. I needed some help getting out of bed - I am not
sure if I twisted myself but my lower back is sore - so Rob was there helping
and the next thing I remember is him telling me to wake up. Wake up? I was

so confused because I was awake - or was I? A little *Twilight Zone* happening in the house of Kenosha (beware if you stay - you too might start fainting).

I guess we all have limits and 2 faints is Rob's. He called 911. I was taken down the stairs in a blanket chair (I am not sure the technical term) and all I could think of was, I need to brush my teeth and get ready. I didn't even have on shoes.

What this outing did was get my friends ready for an emergency - quite the troopers! The kids were taken care of; I had visitors and everything one needs when they are in the ER.

No one would listen when I said I was feeling well and wanted to go home - so I endured a brain scan again (I still have a brain), x-rays-which showed positive for blood clots - very common in cancer patients - but that meant another test (Ct-scan? It was the one with the dye injected in me). Another IV - lots of blood drawn - lots of blood pressure (which was always pretty good - maybe a little low at first) and a night stay at Kenosha's finest! (Not the jail, the hospital.) The people were very kind and really helped move me in a way that hurt as little as possible.

I missed Beeca's best meet, but my brother took over 300 pictures so I was able to see most of the action in still pictures. Rob brought me dinner and I took a nap. Not a bad day I suppose. I slept well - I wasn't hooked up to any machines so I am not sure if they even came in during the night. But as soon as I saw the nurse and the doctor in the morning, I was telling them I wanted to go home.
I was half dressed by the time they let me out. I was able to walk the halls on Sunday morning, so I was leaving my room quite a bit to hang out in the family room. It was nice. My sister-in-law Kristin helped Raney do her homework in the sunroom at the hospital.

When I got home Rob took Raney to go grocery shopping and my 8 yr-old was my babysitter. She would rather have gone out and played with her friends, so I am not sure she is the best choice! Just kidding - we read together.

Raney, Becca, and I started to scrap book our pictures. I always thought I should organize them first but since that is never going to happen, I am just doing pages and maybe those can get organized in some fashion.

I think that I just had a reaction to the chemo - I have a call into the doctor right now so that this won't happen again. I am not sure Rob will be able to take it if it does! The family joke is that he wanted me to clean something and I didn't want to do it, so I fainted and I had to do it twice because the first time didn't get his attention well enough. But two times gets me a trip to the hospital so I might want to clean next time...then again, the paramedics were cute so maybe I will just make sure I look my best next time - JUST KIDDING!! There will be no next time!!!!!

My car needs a jump - Rob will help me out there - but there is no escaping the house of Kenosha without a car, and I am not sure when Rob will get around to that, but I can call USAA Auto club if he takes too long.

Well everyone thanks for listening and thanks for all the help that we received this weekend from family and friends. Have a wonderful, uneventful day, but remember to laugh or do something silly like having a hot fudge sundae for lunch!!!

Until next time take care
Love to all

Posted Sep 29, 2008 10:39am

What is the real culprit behind my fainting? That would be a mix of anesthesia, Benadryl, and Tylenol with codeine - I guess I am a lightweight when it comes to taking drugs. Now I know that I should take one drug at a time and float on that instead of doing more.

I am a free woman - no doctor appointment until Fri. But I probably will see the cavalry (Dr. Fine, Dr. Kaklamani, Gina, Michelle, etc....) Friday. I better be on my best behavior.

Have a good rest of the day. I am getting things done (at the computer - relax people)

See ya soon

Good Morning! I hope everyone is having a great day and enjoying the presence of fall. The leaves are beautiful and I turned on the heat this morning in the car!!

I was driving somewhere in Kenosha and I heard on the radio as I was scanning stations, "I stand up to the Giant". Of course this has created quite the impression on me!

I started to think about all the Giants that the "little people" stand up to every day: bullies, big companies, criminals, etc - and win. So I decided that I should have no problem standing up to my big Giant (cancer) and winning; and one of the main reasons is because of all my family and friends supporting me. So when I have moments, hours, or days of despair and want to fall down and just say NO MORE, my group moves in tightly and I can't fall and my group carries me to my moments, hours, days, weeks, years of laughter, joy, and most of all hope. And of course God is right beside us helping. So anyway, once again a huge THANK YOU. Without the calls, emails, cards, flowers, and prayers, I would be in trouble.

My other random thought is I should start to think more like my children in my outlook of life. Becca asked me on the phone when I was at the hospital "how do you get food, Mama?" and when I told her they bring it to me she said "you're lucky, Mom." And I am lucky; not because they bring me food but because I am able to receive medical care when needed.

Raney claims I am not sick - when I told her that the cancer is back she said "not again, you just had it" My child doesn't see a sick Mom, she just sees me.

118

My mom taught us not to malpractice ourselves and I think that I have taken that to heart because I, like Raney, have a hard time believing I am sick. But my mom also did what the doctors asked of her (she certainly asked the questions to be in control, but she trusted the doctors) and that is what I am going to do. I am going to shock the doctors, like my mom did for many MANY years!!!!!

I am feeling so much better than Saturday and I am remembering what is really important this time around. I don't think that I made enough changes last time, so here is another wake up call to get my priorities straight.

Cancer has given me the opportunity of making my relationships with God, Rob, Raney and Becca, family, friends, stronger, and at the end of the day I'm a much happier person for those gifts. I wouldn't choose cancer - and I certainly wouldn't choose for it to come back - but I can't control that. I can control what I do with this Giant and I am going to come out the WINNER!!!

Have a wonderful day-
Love to all

Posted Oct 3, 2008 3:52pm

In talking with my brother this morning, he was offering a suggestion of doing something fun on my "off" days. I was thinking of emailing the ladies of the neighborhood to see what kind of day we could create together, but that day will have to wait. My white counts were too low so I will be back on Friday to try again for the chemo.

I did meet with the nutritionist with my sister and she said she has a woman who has followed new eating habits and has become a poster child - her blood is so good! So I am signing up to become the 2nd poster child. I don't need to be first, but I want my picture on the wall with a great, big, gold star!!!

I was able to have lunch with my two brothers who work downtown. Larry asked me what my plans were after we had eaten and were walking back to the places we needed to get to and I said "to live". I didn't understand what he was asking. Jimee had to step in and tell him I am having chemo next Friday.

Are you ready for some honesty? I'll wait for some of you to get the Kleenex since I have been told that I am making people cry again. I am getting good at that.

When we were meeting with the nutritionist, she made a comment about having to speak to Karen (the nurse) so I had an idea that she had seen my numbers and knew they were not going to give me chemo. When I finally spoke with Karen and she told me my counts were low and that this was a concern because my numbers dropped quite a bit in the first week (which they don't see too often I guess) I was a bit freaked. When I called Jimee to tell him the news, he asked what that meant and I told him that I am on shaky ground and not feeling very confident. Jimee's perception is the chemo is doing its job and killing the cells. I am back on solid ground but I will be nervous on Friday until I get plugged in. Who knew I would love chemo this much. It keeps me here with you!!

I am going to start the walking club again and I am going to start eating more plant-based foods. I learned today that pork is considered a red meat; and the commercials told me it's the other white meat! Always learning something!!!!

I am mentally better and I am moving forward; I am looking forward to many more years.

Posted Oct 7, 2008 9:15pm

Hello my friends
I am on quite a path and I will tell you I am feeling so blessed and lucky. I can't thank you all enough for the love and the support that I get all the time in prayers, cards, emails, dinners, cleanings, flowers, rides for the family, and so much more.

Cancer: Even though it is a scary thought at times, it has really opened my eyes again to the beauty of this world - with all you wonderful people. This is a great place to be. I am becoming the person I should be and want to be; I am so much happier now. I am eating healthier and feeling so much better. I did a Reiki treatment and it was wonderful. It is like acupuncture but without the needles - energy work. I left feeling light and hopeful. They were saying how fear blocks our energy and that even with a diagnosis of cancer, I can't let fear stop me from living the life I have. I don't know how long I have in this life, but then none of us know that. I don't want fear to rule my day. I want the love and care that I get from God, family and friends to be my direction of living every day.

Raney and I talked about how I can send her love if I am called home to God. I can't remember how the conversation got started, but I told her that I would send her messages in the wind or flowers. She asked how she would know that they were from me and I said she would just know. She said she is hoping that Ceci, Angi, Andrea, and Sarah are getting messages from their parents in some manner.

This is the time for these conversations, while I look and feel healthy. Then I know that I have planted a seed in her brain. Me being a control freak, I have already warned Rob about my haunting him if he does things that I don't like - and Rob wants nothing to do with spirits visiting him. I like harassing him!

I better be off to bed. I hope all of you have a wonderful evening and a great tomorrow. I love life because you are a part of it!!!!

Posted Oct 10, 2008 12:48pm

Patty asked me to post her update; she is on her way back to Wisconsin.

Today did not start out so well. Patty had the chills last night and this morning she became light-headed and dizzy at the train station. The thoughts and prayers to get her white blood cell count up worked, but a little too much. She went from 1.6 to over 18 because she is fighting an infection; so no chemo again today.

Patty was put on oral antibiotics and had blood drawn for another culture. Tomorrow she will get the results and if the infection is in the blood stream she will need to go into the hospital for more aggressive treatment. If the infection is not in the blood stream, then she will stay with the pills.

Patty saw the oncologist today who did not seem overly concerned. She told Patty that they are using an aggressive chemo treatment. The good news is that Patty did not lose any weight from last week. She will try for chemo again next week. Patty says the third time is a charm.

Kristin, my wife, Patty and I had our weekly lunch, and Kristin is going to drive Patty home today, so Patty did not need to take the train all the way to Kenosha.

Patty sends her love and thanks for all the light, prayers and food that have been sent her way.

Jimee

Posted Oct 11, 2008 8:54am

After Patty arrived in Kenosha, her temperature spiked to 102 degrees, so she and Rob dropped off the kids with Lori and headed back to Chicago.

Patty pleased the ER staff by spiking to 103.7 degrees and she kept getting chills. Patty has an infection in her blood stream and they are going to take a CT of her neck to see if there is an infection pocket. Patty will be at Northwestern for a couple of days, with her 42" plasma TV and a view of The Water Tower.

Patty's feeling fine, but she is a bit tired. She did not get into the room until 1:00A.M. They did not have an experienced vampire for Patty, so she was poked and bruised until they had to give up.

Jimee

122

Patty is getting her port removed this morning; they believe that is the sight of the infection. She is hoping to be discharged on Monday, but she was still getting the chills yesterday.

Patty was given a very large care package from Equinox yesterday. Rob was too nervous to leave the room, so he ate a power bar designed for women. (He liked it so much he may get some for later!) Patty told Becca that she was given a large box of Lemonheads and Becca told her she was so lucky.

While Kristin and I were visiting, Rob went down to get a couple of drinks. He was gone for a very long time and Patty was wondering why he was taking so long. He came back with some chocolate from Ghirardelli's. What he did not realize was how crowded it gets on the weekend and it is marathon weekend in Chicago. He and Patty decided that there was to be no more weekend visits to Northwestern.

The girls are staying with Lori and Carrie this weekend, so it is just Rob and Patty in Chicago.

Hopefully Patty will have access to a computer and can begin adding her own blogs again.

Thank you again for your kind words and prayers.

Jimee

Posted Oct 13, 2008 9:24am

Patty spent her first night alone at the hospital and survived.

She still needs to be infection free before she can have the pic line put in. Her port was removed yesterday morning, with no complications. She was then sent back to her room where she and Rob watched football on her 42" T.V. Rob went home after the Bears game and Katy came to visit. Patty was

123

able to see the photo albums that I downloaded: one of her birthday, one of Becca's gymnastics meet, and one of her nephew's soccer game. We were able to watch it on the big TV.

Patty still does not have a departure date or time. She's been enjoying her lunch and dinners, but the breakfasts aren't so hot, literally. Saturday she ordered tilapia for dinner, but forgot that she was in a hospital and not a restaurant. All she got was a 4 oz piece of fish, no rice, no vegetables. She and Rob laughed at the food. But it was so good she ordered it again on Sunday, but added her vegetables. Her temperature is gone, and she has not lost any weight.

Patty is getting tired of getting poked. This is not like the acupuncture that she enjoys so much.
She is expecting her father, husband, and two brothers today for visitors. They are going to do a test for Patty to see if she has an infection in her heart. If that is the case, then she will be on antibiotics for 4 weeks instead of the 12 days regiment that she is currently on. The 12 days begin when the first culture comes back negative.

Jimee

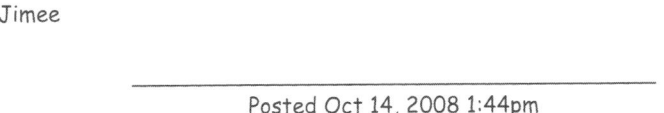

Posted Oct 14, 2008 1:44pm

Patty has one more test and then she is free, unfortunately, the test is not until 3:00 and she needs to meet with the home-care nurse before 5:00 in Kenosha to learn how to take her antibiotics. It looks like Wednesday morning she will be departing the Windy City for home, for a return visit on Friday for Chemo Round II Session II. Patty has been trying to get this chemo for 3 weeks, but as the Doctor pointed out, Patty is only 1 week behind (due to the off week).

She is having a difficulty remaining positive. Yesterday was one of her bad days; today is not as bad. Patty's suggestion for the day: if you ever find yourself in the hospital and you like your children, bring pictures, recordings, and locks of hair with you. If you can get away with it, take their blanket as well. Patty is ready to begin fighting the cancer; she is fed up with fighting the infection.

Tuesdays at Northwestern are special days at the Prentice Hospital for the patients on the chemo floor. Imagine a very long Q-tip, about 5" that does not go into your ear and it hurts to sit down for awhile.

Please keep sending the kind words and thoughts. Patty's sister Katy sent an e-mail that caused Patty to laugh so hard Rob was worried she would hurt herself.

Jimee

While it was true that Patty only had one test to go before she was to be released, her test was not considered an emergency and there were too many of those so she was bumped. She still has one test left.

She was almost transferred to the prison wing, after being starved for 6 hours before the "test", then she was visited by a doctor and a nurse. Luckily there was nothing for Patty to throw at them.

The new plan is for her is to "fast" again tomorrow and then she will be released after her last antibiotic cocktail, which is around 10:00pm. SEND THE LIGHT - SHE NEEDS TO GO HOME!!!!!!
Thursday morning: she learned how to hook up her IV at 6:30am.

On a lighter note, Patty was parenting from Chicago, telling Raney to do her homework and call her when she was finished so that Raney can play the clarinet for her. A few minutes after she hung up, while Patty was talking to her sister, her cell phone rang - it was from her house. Patty kept talking to her sister, and ignored the 9 calls from home. Patty thought that Raney had a silly question, but when Patty called back, she was connected to a distraught daughter - Valentine had left Raney a "present" on her bedroom floor. The miniature dachshund had killed another miniature hamster. Valentine: 2, Hamsters: 0.

125

Grandpa says that he needs a new contract; dealing with dead carcasses was not in the original agreement. If Patty is not released tomorrow, Carrie, bring the van around back and we will break her out of this joint.

Jimee

Rob has been fired. He failed to find the good stuff in the hospital. While Patty and I were watching the 42" "boob" tube, we started playing with the internet. When we called this place the "spa", we did not realize they give foot and hand massages - but we'd missed it.

Cancel the escape plan; Patty is staying until she gets her massage. Tomorrow is the Jolly Trolley. Monday she missed bedside Bingo. On our most recent tour of the penthouse floor, Patty found a "family" room, an overnight room with 2 beds. Now the girls can stay too. We just need to find someone with no small animals to watch the killer dog.

Patty has a gabby nurse tonight, John. He told her that she had the good staph infection, not the resistant kind - that is the kind that is resistant to the antibiotics. Good thing we were able to play in the fields as kids and not worry about that entire anti-bacterial gunk. Patty's immune system is very strong.

The girls are getting a little worried that Patty is not coming home. It is kind of weird that she's still in the hospital because she was too healthy to get the test she needed to leave. Becca understood that logic.

Patty is getting a little punchy; we are taking this journey one day at a time, but these healthy days spent in the hospital are getting a little ridiculous. No fever, blood pressure back to normal and the blood is clear.
For those of you who are reading this Tuesday evening: Go to bed! The rest of you - good morning.

Jimee

They are telling Patty that she is "definitely" on the list to have her test done, and they are planning to give her the antibiotics "early" tonight so that she can head north, for a full day and a half, so she can come back south on Friday to get her overdue chemo treatment.

Pedal pulses good, blood pressure good, temp good. It is 9:20am, Patty should be released in about 12 hours but she is already dressed and ready to go. I (Jimee) cannot imagine what will happen on the 16th floor if Patty does not get discharged today.

I'm sure she will begin saying her goodbyes to the staff in about 4 hours so that she is ready to go at 9:30 tonight.

Will keep you posted.

Jimee

Let's give Jimee a great big thanks and cheer!!! I wasn't sure that he would want to turn over the reins but he did so with only a little kicking and screaming - nothing that would embarrass him too much. Jimee was my night nurse so that Rob was able to go home to Raney and Becca.

OK. My last day was long with the TTR (I think that is the name of the test to see if I have an infection in my heart). I don't think I complain too much, but let me tell you - after being poked without any success in the ER room, getting my port taken out - while I was awake so I was able to see all the fun tools, getting a pic line that made me scream a couple of times and have a few tears of pain, and being locked in my hospital room for 5 days - I wasn't the happiest patient about yet another test - especially one that was delayed.

The heart test requires one to have their throat numb. I am not sure what kind of person discovers and invents the most disgusting tasting gel medicine but they are very good at their job! I have never tasted anything so gross in my entire life and will not be repeating this test. I had to put a Popsicle stick with this gel junk in my mouth. I almost threw up. Then I wasn't able to swallow, because the medicine did its job and I was numb, only to wait too long for the doctor (he was in another procedure and the nurse misjudged the timing of his completion) so I was no longer numb. Then I tried this thick liquid disgusting stuff that numbed the lips so back to the gel. Thank God I hadn't eaten anything all day or I would have thrown up. Then I got sprayed three times by opening my mouth and holding my breath and then breathing out - no numbing in the lungs, breathing is a good thing. I was then put out and I don't remember the camera going down my throat. The nurse used Raney and Becca as incentives to get me to gargle the thick liquid when I told them I wasn't sure that I could do this anymore.

Lesson # 204: Don't tell the nurses how desperate you are to go home - they turn on you and make you gargle gross thick liquids. (She was very nice and she didn't really turn on me.)

I survived and Rob and I made it home around 10:30pm, I think. I had a smile on my face the whole way home. Northwestern is a fine facility and I am happy that places like that are available to me, but this was way too long to be gone. I walked the dog tonight as the kids got ready for bed and I felt like I have been gone a month. The trees have changed a lot, Raney and Becca are seven inches taller, and someone named Joey keeps calling to take Raney out on a date. My babies are growing up so fast. I am just kidding - they were right back to teasing each other and wanting my attention. I love being home.

Today the home nurse dropped off a pharmacy at our house-

I will have to get back to you ... medicine time.

OK, so now I have a pharmacy in my upstairs closet and my refrigerator. Rob, Carrie and I were given a crash course in how to push drugs into my veins - Carrie and I had no problems but Rob (did I tell you what a nervous ninny he is?) went completely white every time I moved. I just giggled a lot - I am my mother's daughter.

Well, it's late and I am tired-

My day was great and I really enjoyed my freedom!!! Even though my last blog seemed like I went through the wringer, I really only had one moment of really hard time because I was really missing my kids. Poke me, gag me, put cameras down my throat, but don't keep me from my children.

The whole staff at NW was so kind; I was really starting to feel like I was getting to know some of them. I was even starting rumors with Kristin (my sister-in-law).

Sleep tight and talk to you later

Back to Chicago for the really good drugs; the stuff at home is small potatoes compared to Chicago!

I am not taking the train. Rob is taking me this time. I am not sure when he is going to leave my side – oh, that would be Sunday for a Bears game. Nothing gets in the way of a game (and I am just kidding, Rob has missed a few games to be with me).

Good night

I know that I am a bit behind in my updates so let's get started. As you all know, I came home Wednesday night with a huge a** smile on my face. Thurs. morning was pretty much like another - after the nurse showed up with the pharmacy - but Rob drove the girls to school (or my neighbor picked them up. I can't remember now).

Rob and the doctor discussed my driving when I got home without me being in the room, and it was determined that I shouldn't drive for a couple of days. Rob is way too paranoid - I mean, what's a couple of hospital visits. I don't think that should get his undies in a bunch (or whatever that saying is). Rob wouldn't let me walk the hallways without someone being with me, but as soon as I got home I was free to go grocery shopping with a friend. Of course, we went out to lunch with another friend first. After what seemed like a month, it was great to get out with some of the ladies and have a real meal. The hospital food was not bad, but after 13 meals I had had enough. (Rob did get us pizza one time and Indian food that was soooooooooo good!!)

Thursday I was out and about, getting the house back to normal, catching up on laundry, going through the mail - all the important things I do. I did it all with help from friends and my dad.

Let me tell you that Rob is a rule-bound Reggie (old video arts people should recognize this phrase). We asked the nurse about the antibiotic schedule and how strict it needed to be and she said that you can take it 1/2 hr in either direction, but Rob will not let me get the medicine early so I can't go to bed before 10:30pm. He makes us get up at 5:30am to get the medicine out of the refrigerator (we were told that if we don't take the medicine out of the refrigerator the patient - that would be me - would get chilled because the medicine is injected rather close to the heart; and I want no chillin'- well maybe if I am having a hot flash!!).

Anyway the medicine is going pretty well but I will be happy when it is done so I can get back to sleeping in until 6:30am on school days. I will be done on Sat!!!!

Thursday is done and Rob and I get up Friday to go back downtown for the chemo. I am now getting the shot that I had last year to boost my white blood counts, but let me tell you, when I was hooked up again I was very restless. I had just spent 5 days being hooked up to the IV three times a day for about 1 hr each time and I just didn't want to be attached anymore. I had to stand during some of the chemo. This time was a bit shorter and the next time will even be shorter. I am now going every other week (which means on Halloween Rob and the girls will be with me (they don't have school) so we might do something afterwards in the city that is Halloweenie!!

I will get the Avastin and the Gemzar together now so Jimee's original report has been completely changed - I hope you people are able to go with the flow. Thank God I come from a big family who have no problem rolling with the punches - as long as there are no needles involved or gross gel numbing stuff or yanking out the port, or my least favorite, getting the pic line.

After chemo, Rob and I stopped in Kenosha for Rob to get his hair cut, and I went to Kohl's to look for socks for Raney and Becca. (I was allowed to walk the store alone until Rob was finished!!! I am a free woman now.)

The weekend was nice. My brother, Larry, my nephew, Aidan (who is turning three 10/25), and my sister, Katy, came to visit me. The girls went to a Brownie thing and I just hung out. The group of us went to a Silpada Jewelry party - which Aidan loved because there were lots of kids. Katy and I left with Larry and Aidan. Rob and the girls came home in time for me to get my medicine. Rob has really been good about this even though I harass him about not going a half hour early.

Now Monday: I was able to sign up for a free facial from a spa in Kenosha - Arvasi (they offered a day for cancer patients) - and let me tell you, it was so wonderful. I almost thought I was too tired to go but I decided against that and I am so happy. I was given a paraffin wax on the hands and a scalp massage - I was in heaven. They have a great relaxation room; local Kenoshans, you should go (and no I wasn't paid to advertise). I don't remember the rest of the day, but does anyone after a real spa visit??

Now it is Tuesday and I am feeling the effects of the shot. If I remember correctly it messes with my bone marrow and makes my bones hurt - and it is working well! What does one do when their bones ache? They take their prima donna dog for a walk to the lake. Valentine is a hard one to walk seeing how she has to sniff everything and bark at all the big dogs and people. But the lake was beautiful today; some waves and blue skies. What more could I ask for?

I am tired and I want to go to bed, but I have to wait for the right time to get my medicine. There will be no medicine before its time!

I think I forgot to tell you, I read *Son of a Witch* (the book after *Wicked*) and I really enjoyed it.

Overall I am doing well and finding the silver lining in all things. I'm also going to Reiki. I am going to try yoga this week and am learning to find the inner peace in my body. I am gathering information to send to a nutritionist in UT that was written in a book and helped a brain tumor person keep his cancer at bay for over 12 years.

I am doing it all this time around. This time is very loud and clear that I need to change things and take myself to the next level. I can eat flaxseeds for the rest of my life and have dark chocolate - I don't mind. I want to suffer through Raney's teen years just like my mother did with me - Payback Baby!! And let me tell you, Raney is already practicing and she is good (I think better than I was.)

good night, sleep tight.

Please keep the prayers going. I told Rob that it is my turn to shock the doctors (when I get scanned again - I don't know when that is yet) I am done with them shocking me!!!!!

Talk to you later
Lots of love and pamper yourself next month - you deserve it.

Posted Oct 22, 2008 9:16pm

I was telling someone that there is a silver lining in everything - and the silver lining to getting my medicine at 10:00pm is acting like an adult! I am staying up later than the kids so I have time to do some adult things. Now if I wasn't on the medicine I could think of a few bottles that I would be hitting about this time. Maybe next week; I will have to see if I can handle drugs and alcohol. (Remember, this is red ribbon week so I have to say no this week but next week is a whole new story).

I forgot to mention that my niece, Nea, came over last night and we went and got Raney and Becca their Halloween costumes. Becca is going to be a bumblebee and Raney is going to be a ladybug. My little insects!!! Rob is going to be Elton John - I think he liked the flashy gold sunglasses and went from there - and I am not sure what I am going to be, but I am sure that there is something from the attic I can find. I missed the opportunity last year to be Uncle Fester, and I am not shaving my head (yet); maybe someday, when I am donating for some worthy case but not for candy that I shouldn't be eating anyway.

Today my sister-in-law came over and we were working on a webpage. I am creating a career for me to do out of the house since I have to keep saying no to subbing (no to drugs, alcohol and subbing, that is my motto) so I was busy with that until the kids came home and then it was all about them.

I did walk the dog down to the lake to get my exercise and my peaceful time. I had to get on the fast track so I can learn to slow down and lead a less stressful life. I am in a hurry to slow down; what a good slogan for something out there.

I might go over to the yoga tomorrow and see what that is all about - probably something I should have tried years ago. But it is never too late to try something new.

I remember what I wanted to let you know: Take a day off and do something fun with a friend, spouse, kids, and siblings - don't wait for the tomorrows. I am not saying do this every day, but if there is a movie or a museum exhibit go and make memories when it isn't super crowded and remember how fun it was to play hooky. (Now Dad, I didn't play hooky, people just told me how much fun it was.)

I was really bummed that I wasn't able to take Raney and Becca out of school for Columbus day (I think that I need to get over the hospital visit now), and I am going to take them out soon just to play games all day and maybe have ice cream for lunch!!!

I can't remember what the other silver linings that I found were, but if I remember them I will let you know. Amongst the bad there is good somewhere; I just need to keep remembering that. I am not afraid to ask God for a pardon this time around. I have a lot to do and I am rearing to go. Every day I wake up I am thanking God for a wonderful day - and if I yell at the kids I just try to do better on the next day.

Thanks for all the comments. I don't know how to respond to them individually like before, but I do read them all and am truly touched by all your thoughts and prayers. I have a few new people, so welcome to the gabby room. I am a rambler, aren't I? But my typing is getting much better! (Told you - a silver lining everywhere.)

Love to all and may your dreams be sweet and not one of needles trying to find you to poke and poke.

Posted Oct 23, 2008 9:46pm

Oops, well you all know by now how anal my husband is about me taking the medicine at the 6:00am, 2:00pm, and 10:00pm marks with not a minute to spare. Tonight I went to take out my dose for the 10:00pm injection when I realized there are none left which means I have no antibiotics for my 6:00am injection! So of course the sirens are going off in Rob's head and I made a call to Walgreens and the earliest I will get my medicine is about 9:00am (the lengths I go through just to sleep in!!!!). I am sure that it isn't going to send me back to the spa of Chicago, but that is a chance Rob really doesn't want to take.

Today was a good day. I took the pup down to the lake (I am not sure she liked it too much - it was a bit windy) and I sat on the beach and I imagined God filling me up with perfect cells that squeeze out the bad ones which I sent back to God for Him to heal.

On the radio I heard this woman talking about her near death experience where she saw herself from above. She was talking about when you die, the only thing that matter is the love you received and gave and how you feel about yourself. Then my radio turned to static on me so I didn't get the rest of the story.

134

I thought that was pretty good advice (but I think that I am also supposed to enjoy this planet - it is a wonderful place to live and I still get amazed every time I see Lake Michigan which has such personality).

I am going to get ready for bed; I am tired tonight.
Talk to you later and have a wonderful day.

Remember to love and be loved! I am blessed by all of you and I am able to grow in the love area - a great place to be! Life is wonderful when there is love everywhere.
lol

The eagle has flown the coop: Rob has left the building!!!!!!!!!!

OK, I need to back up a bit. As you remember, I didn't have my medicine for the morning so I was able to sleep in until 6:30am!!!!! and both the pharmacist and the nurse said to make the 2nd dose a bit later but that I could stay on the 10pm push. However, no one bothered to tell Rob so he had me up until 10:30pm. One way or another I am not able to sleep during "treatment". Take me back to the hospital; they were so good that when they unplugged me I stayed asleep!! Just kidding. I am becoming like Dorothy, "there is no place like home. There is no place like home. There is no place like home." I just don't think I would do well in the glittery red shoes; not my style. On the last day of antibiotics Rob quit his nursing job so I am on my own again. (I rehire him for about 6 minutes to flush the tube at night; but that can be done at anytime to keep the tubes clean. I will not wear dirty tubes!!!)

I have survived the antibiotics. I am not sure when they are going to take blood (vampire season, I better watch out on how much they take this week) to make sure all the "bugs" are out of my system. But I am feeling great.

We went trick-or-treating on Sunday, but by 5:00pm I needed to go in. I was freezing and, luckily, so were my children. Dressing them up as flappers was one of my better ideas this year - especially with no coats! But people needed to see the dresses. I am kidding. Raney and Becca were insects - Raney was a ladybug and Becca was a bumble bee. I was thinking of going as a fainting patient so that Rob could follow me and call 911 every block or two. Or I was thinking about being a runaway patient with my tube hanging from my arm as I scream, "please, no more drugs!" It would have gone well with "Just say no to drugs" week. I ended up being a dead bride; and Rob told me how great I looked! I had on makeup and did my hair. Isn't it wonderful that my husband likes the "dead" look? I will have to say I am not sure what he thinks about the black nail polish so maybe there is still hope??

There was something else I wanted to share but now I can't remember it. I probably should have gone as a zombie since I don't think they have brains.

Friday I go for Chemo and Raney and Becca don't have school so we are going to dress up for the treatment and have some fun. I can't go as the dead bride (won't Rob be upset) because they won't be able to get to the tube, so I have to think of a whole new costume. Luckily my spa appointment isn't until 12:15pm, so we don't have to leave at the crack of dawn on an off day. I have been hearing that it is supposed to be nice this weekend!!! I am staying out of the hospital for this weekend - I love Indian summer.

Now I remember what I was going to share with you. Rob asked me to take his clothes to the cleaners then asked when the last time I went to the cleaners was. I can't remember yesterday, so there is no way I am going to be able to remember that. You would think with that comment that he had a truck load to go, right? Two pair of pants - that is the load. And he comes downstairs in a sports jacket and jeans. So, of course, I said a smart a** comment.

My arm doesn't hurt anymore from the pic, and the vein that was thoroughly tortured is starting to feel a whole lot better. I am on the mend! I am sending all the bad cells to God and I am feeling wonderful.

Remember how I said there is a silver lining in everything? Sometimes I can't find it, but I am getting chemo again and have a pic line during fall. I don't have to rake or pick up leaves or snow blow when the snow hits, and I was able to wear a bathing suit this summer. See, I am no dummy.

To be honest I didn't need a second time around. I would have raked leaves and been happy to do so. Now I will just make warm apple cider and hot chocolate and call it a day.

I was told that I either make my readers laugh or cry; funny how that works. When I am tired, I think I make you cry; when I have lots of energy, I think I make you laugh. It is good to get in touch with a range of emotions, and laughter and tears is a great range. I have been told that my meds must be off because I am getting mushy. Mushy comes when I start calling and telling you how important you are to me and that I love you. Now that is ultimate mushy!!!! I might make you cry though, so are you ready????

Have a wonderful day. I need to play the role of Cinderella before her prince comes and rescues her: mopping, vacuuming, laundry, dishes, beds, bathrooms...the list is endless.

I am kidding, but I do have a few things to do.
Love to all

Posted Oct 30, 2008 12:36pm

The kids are off school today and tomorrow so I thought it would be fun to make a pumpkin pie and apple pie for the staff on the 21st floor - I even got them scary plates.

I am trying to figure out what a good costume would be for tomorrow since the dead bride covers my arm too well and no one would be able to plug me - unless I decided to be a stripper!!!

Driving around Kenosha and Chicago land we see construction all the time, so I was thinking I could be a construction sign: "Boobs under Construction".

But I will not be a fainting patient on the 21st floor; too close to a real room and I am not checking in again!!! (Am I still harboring bad feeling about my hospital stay??? They were very nice so that wasn't the problem. It's just that if I am going to be gone for 5 days, I want to be on the sunny beaches of Mexico).

I am under the impression that even if the white counts are low I will still get chemo because of the shot on Saturday.

One more thing and then I need to go. Raney, Becca and I were downstairs going through winter clothes (UUGH!!!!!) and I opened up a tub that is holding things from my childhood and Raney and Becca's infancy. I still have a teddy bear I was given for my 10th b-day (I was in 5th grade) and Raney wanted to show it to Becca. As she went running upstairs she was screaming, "Becca, I got something cool to show you. It's so OLD!" Wasn't that nice of my sweetie?? She wants me to give it to her for her 5th grade b-day and then she will give it to Becca - a new family tradition. I am not sure what will happen to it once Becca has her birthday though.

I am feeling great and have pretty good energy until about 8:00ish. Thankfully that is when the kids are close to bedtime.

I really appreciate all the prayers and everything. I believe that is why I am feeling so good--
Enjoy the weather

Posted Nov 2, 2008 10:51am

I called the PA before my treatment on Friday to ask about the flu shot and a blood test to compare my omega 3 vs. omega 6. She didn't call back but stopped in to see me instead - with the flu shot. Last year I didn't get it, but I am a little more paranoid of germs these days. I grimaced at the thought of the flu shot, but it didn't hurt at all. My friend who gives me my shot, to help with the white counts, went out of town for a wedding this weekend. I had to give the shot to myself because Nurse Rob doesn't like needles (I don't think he is going to pass his medical degree). Rob wanted me to wait for someone else to be able to do it. I, on the other hand, want to give my white counts all the help they need to stay in the right range so I am able to fight off infections that are looming everywhere; I just can't see them. It wasn't as bad as I thought. I was a bit nervous to shoot myself, but I do what I need to do. I have endurance and strength from meditation!!! Sometimes my endurance is a bit behind what I would like; then I take a nap.

138

I think all the flu shot did was make me not feel well yesterday. I was in bed by 6:30pm and Rob took the girls to see High School Musical 3. I slept until 8:30ish, put on my PJs, brushed my teeth and went back to bed. The girls were really good (they even had a couple of friends over) and I really didn't hear much from them until about 6:00AM (darn this time change). I will be messed up all day with how early it is.

I had a print-out of my orders and I am getting Avistin until the end of Nov, Gemzar at the beginning of Jan, and Zometa through Aug. Once I am on Zometa only, I will only need to go downtown once a month for a 15 infusion. Maybe then I will be allowed back on the train??? I bought a 10 ride that I need to use in a year's time. See how strong I believe myself to be??

Backing up a bit, I went to meditation yesterday morning and during our visualization the woman, Joyce, made a comment about how we get completely new cells every 9 months. So that is my goal. I picture the perfect cells multiplying and the bad ones squeezing out of my body. I would prefer this to happen before nine months, so we will have to wait and see if that miracle comes my way.

And my goal this week is to get to at least one yoga class.

The other thing I did was order *Faulty Towers* from the library. If you haven't seen these I highly recommended them. John Cleese is in them and they are so funny. I told a friend that I was going to have a laughing hour with the ladies of Kenosha, and we are going to ripple laughter throughout Kenosha and beyond. I tried to get *Soap* (with Billy Crystal) but the library didn't have them. That's also very funny.

Some of my family is coming over today. We are starting a Silly Sunday where we play cards or a board game; something to get us laughing. I made 2 pumpkin pies and an apple pie for the festivities (with ice cream of course).

Well I better get ready for the family.

I hope you all had a great weekend. I am feeling tired but I think by Tuesday all will be good again.

What a day
Posted Nov 4, 2008 1:43pm

I woke up to "The Drive" - Journey was playing (still one of my favorite bands) and it wasn't pitch black outside! So many plusses already, and it only gets better...

Becca slept with me last night. Raney and Aunt Katy (who tried to go home yesterday but I kidnapped her as she politely tells anyone who will listen) slept downstairs. So after my shower I was singing and dancing for Becca (I even made her smile which is no small feat with that child in the morning), and I was singing down the laundry chute for Katy and Raney to join in on the beauty of the day. Now, Katy tells me I scared the dog but I don't believe that. I think she just wanted to get home and thought being mean about my lovely singing voice would make me send her on her merry way.

And because I sang so lovely Becca made me breakfast.

After dropping the girls off at school, Katy and I went for tea/coffee with a friend and, oops, Katy missed the last morning train out of Kenosha. But how does one leave the coffee house as we are sitting OUTSIDE in Nov??? We did eventually leave, and I then went and voted in the historic election of my lifetime. What a wonderful day to be alive! The trees are on fire in Kenosha; it's perfect weather; and 35 years ago my baby brother was born (HAPPY BIRTHDAY RYAN!!!!). I remember the phone call when we were told Ryan joined us; what an impact to remember something that long ago when I can't remember 2 minutes ago most of the time (chemo brain must only effect short term memory). So, Ryan, I am telling you publicly that you are an important part of my life (as are all my family and friends).

No, I am not hitting the vodka and I am off medicines. I just love Indian summer. It does a body good!!! (And being mushy can be so much fun!! You should try it today.)

Now the big question is: will there be days like this in Feb???? Yes, I do believe so as everyday is a gift and I go to bed thanking the Lord above for each day. (And then I ask for more) I am greedy but I have so many plans left for this planet, and Heaven will always be there for us.

Well I, and my energy, need to get a few things done before the girls get home.

So thank you my friends for listening to my rambles and for sending prayers - that does a soul good.
Love to all

Do you feel that I am a step or two behind in updating you??? I am hoping to stop playing the catch up game and get back on track with my friends. Last time I wrote was a good day.

But let's back up to Wednesday. Raney and Becca got out of school at 11:00am (I am not sure why these school days exist but they do) and the weather was very nice. I wanted the girls to help with raking for a couple of hours and then they were going to be allowed to play. If you want to be forced to slow down in your life call my 8 yr-old to help with your raking. Talk about being forced to have patience (Rob worked out of the house and he came outside and told me to not even open the brown bags that the leaves go in).

So to make a long raking story short, Raney and Becca never made it to a play date. We went down to the neighbor's that have 19 month and 2 month old girls. I was taking Raney and Becca to the park and wanted to see if Camryn (19 month) could come with us. The mom, Katie, said yes and asked me to hold the baby, Darby, while she got Camryn ready. I jokingly said that Katie could go to the park with the girls; I was going to stay and hold Darby. Katie jumped on that idea so I was able to get my baby fix - and a nap. I fell asleep holding the baby. When I told Rob he couldn't believe I fell asleep holding a baby; how quickly he forgets that is what I did with the girls all the time.

So Wednesday the universe slowed me down.

141

I will have to finish catching up with you later, I need to get ready for the girls.

So the story continues...
Thanks for listening...

Posted Nov 11, 2008 11:17am

So today is Tuesday and I am not sure if I will be writing about things that haven't happen, have happened, or are going to happen. Maybe I should drink only the finest of the red wines?????

I think I ended last Wednesday, wait, no, I didn't, but I am bringing you back to the morning of Wednesday when Raney and Becca were arguing over something (all the arguments sound the same) so I took the dog for a walk...

One of my favorite things about fall is when the leaves fall like shadows on the ground and are left undisturbed. There were three neighbors in a row who hadn't started to rake so it looked like the sun was on the ground on the cloudy day.

Even with that start, I had a mentally rough day; I am not sure why (I certainly hope that it wasn't due to the clouds or I am in for a rough winter (unless I move to FL for the season!!!).

The day was so bad at one point that I couldn't even look at Raney. I was afraid that I would start to sob and never stop, leaving my 10 yr-old a bit confused. But then when I got to gymnastics, another mom was telling me how hard the day was for her and I was so relieved (not because she was having a bad day, just because I wasn't the only one). As I was getting the kids ready for bed, my baby brother (and we all know his age now) called to let me know that when I give left-over apple pie that will be warmed in the microwave, not to put it on a plate that starts a fire in 22 seconds. Not only was Ryan one call away from 911 (which would have happened in my house as we all know how trigger happy Rob is with 911) but he wasn't able to enjoy the apple pie - oops!!! And then I watched some *Faulty Towers*. My day ended up well!!!!!!

142

Saturday night my dad came and babysat for Raney and Becca. Rob and I went to a fundraiser for the Cancer Wellness Center from Northbrook. This was the place that Raney raised money for in April.

We were treated to a red carpet as we walked into the restaurant, with our choice of red/white wine, champagne, or martinis. At least 100 people were working this event (the restaurant's opening day was Nov 10th so this was also a preview for the community). Every time you turned around there was food or alcohol available. There were 3 ice sculptures, crab legs, oysters on the half shell, ahi tuna, filet mignon sandwiches, lamb with a dill sauce, cheeses, cold cuts, beautiful desserts, some lobster pate', fruits, and live music; all at no cost to the center. They were expecting 500 people. Rob and I spent an evening like the rich and famous. It was a very nice time, but I am turning a bit like a man! The attire was cocktail or business so there were a lot of black dresses and a LOT of boobies!!!

I wanted to grab some of them I thought they looked so good! And as I am having these most inappropriate thoughts about my "sisters", Rob made a comment about all the cleavage. I just had to agree with him - no reprimanding him with my brain going down the same path. But rest assured, I didn't grab anyone. Good thing I am not drinking that much anymore. I stayed with the wine and just looked at the martinis.

Sunday Becca had a meet and then we went for pizza. I fell asleep on the way home so the girls and I were sent to bed at 7:15pm. We watched *Faulty Towers* together first. (I think I should be able to set my own bedtime - so there!!!)

Monday I went to Reiki and they are so kind there. Joyce, who does the treatments, told me at the end of the session that I am to go every Monday until she tells me not to go. She said she felt toxins in my right shoulder area. I forgot to ask if that could be the stuff that I am flushing the pic out with. The people there use the phrase "release the disease you think you have" not the "disease you have". They have a very healthy attitude. I am made in the image of God; a perfect healthy person.

Joyce told me that my mind changes (so I have different colors showing up) a lot so I have some practice ahead of me.

I love that way of thinking. I was given the "homework" of sweeping out any pain with a blue broom. Then I fill myself with green (healing color). I will tell you that I went to bed last night more peaceful than I ever remember. I am going to Reiki every week I am able to go.

Today is a good day; I think my fears are at bay. I think once the scan is done, I will feel more relaxed. The scans are supposed to be early Dec.; a great Christmas present when I get to shock the doctors!!!!

Friday is chemo and the pic will be leaving the body!!!!!!!!!!!! I am so excited, I danced this morning. The port will be put back in Dec. 1 so I have a couple of weeks off - YEAHHHHHHH!!!

Rob would like me to spend the night in the hospital after getting the port. He doesn't forget, does he? I will not be spending the night, but I did promise him that I will not be taking any other drugs then what they give me at the hospital. But if I do fall again, he better wait a couple of hours before calling 911. That is all I have to say on that subject.

We are all caught up. See what happens when Rob works out of the house and I have no phone?

I hope all of you have a wonderful day.

Thanks for listening and I will chat again soon.
Love to all

Posted Nov 17, 2008 10:38am

Just a quickie as I need to get a couple things done today.

My numbers were good on Friday so I was able to get chemo. A friend drove me because I am not allowed on the train anymore. We stopped at Trader Joes on the way to the hospital. The 2nd best part of the day was the pic

144

line was removed!!! (And it didn't hurt at all to remove which was nice since the pain of getting one was clearly a 100 on a scale of 1-10.)

The best part of the day was celebrating the removal of the pic by sharing a chocolate fondue with a friend and my sister. Now I think that would be a great tradition that we should all start this year. At some point during the holiday order a chocolate fondue (much more fun than shopping)!!!

On the way home, my friend and I stopped at an opening for an art gallery in Kenosha - some really nice pieces!!

Saturday was a bit rough. I was very tired and had nausea galore!! I tried to take a nap but Raney kept coming upstairs every 20 minutes to see if I needed anything or how was I feeling. (I am so glad that I didn't have the energy to get mad at her because I found out later that it was Rob sending her upstairs; him I can get mad at.) We now have new rules in the house when I am trying to take a nap after chemo.

I got my shot to keep the white cells behaving. Rob took the girls to a movie and I had some quiet time by myself.

Sunday was a much better day and today is great as well.

We are leaving Sunday for Thanksgiving up in the North woods (where it is snowing!!).
Everyone have a wonderful day, and if I don't get a chance to blog again, Happy Thanksgiving!!!!

I meet Jesus
Posted Nov 19, 2008 12:51pm

I bet your curiosity is peaked, but let me give you some background first. I was born into a Catholic family, and I am raising Raney and Becca with the Catholic beliefs. So basically God and Jesus have always been a part of my life.

Fast forward to a couple years ago. I used to watch this show on Friday nights called *Joan of Arcadia* and I loved the show. In a nutshell it was about a teenage girl who promised God she would do anything if her brother survived a car accident. So He took her up on the offer and would appear to her as a person of different ages, sex, race, wealth, etc., and give her difficult assignments.

Now we are back to Monday, Nov 15th. I went to Reiki and told Joyce that I have never had so much peace inside. After my session she said that my charkas (energy sources) were wide open which is really good because I am receiving God's healing light through my energy sources. So it was another good session. I will miss the next two though because we will be out of town for one and I will be getting chemo the Monday after Thanksgiving.

Now we come to yesterday (don't you just love time travel???).

Rob asked me to get his oil changed in the car so we are ready to drive to Northern WI. When I came home the dog started to bark and Rob quickly asked me to walk her because he was on an important call.

Valentine and I went down to the lakefront and I sat on my bench and said my prayers. I have never said so many formal prayers in my life; I say them with the kids, throughout the day and before I go to bed. Let me tell you, God is showing me He is listening.

As I was turning to go back home a man asked me if I had seen a black glove. I said no and offered the suggestion that if he walked the same path tomorrow he probably would find it. I figured he needed to get somewhere because he was in his car. I was walking back and the man parked his car and yelled something I couldn't hear that well. He got out of his car and yelled something again. So I asked, are you talking to me? He said yes. He had a Frisbee and asked if I would throw it. (He was probably in his late 50s.) I said that I needed to get a few things done before the kids got home from school. (This is where I heard the message) he said, "Don't rush through life; you will miss things."
(I know God has been trying to slow me down; who else would send an 8 yr-old to rake leaves?? I am not sure what is much slower than that?)

So I played Frisbee for about 15 min. Then I told him I needed to go because I was hungry - and I was. I was starting to get a little lightheaded, and we all know what happens if something happens to me while walking the dog. The man said he would feed me. Now I am not going to take food from someone I don't know, so I politely said no. As I was walking home I thought about *Joan of Arcadia* and I realized that person could have been Jesus telling me to slow down and that He will take care of my hunger for peace and health. Then, of course, the Irish-Catholic kicked in and I was scared that I got a bad mark because I walked away from Jesus. See the power of Irish-Catholic guilt???

In talking with my sister, Jesus understands that I am new to this and He won't be offended that I walked away to go eat lunch. Jesus is always there for us.

Can you tell that I am feeling great?

As much as I am supposed to slow down, I do need to take care of the dog because the kids get out of school an hour early. Breathe deep and invite the energy of the planet in....

Posted Nov 22, 2008 10:20pm

Hello my friends!

We are leaving tomorrow for our Thanksgiving trip up North. The girls (and Rob and I) are very excited because there are a few things that we do every year that they really enjoy (and I think they really like eating the pies that they help make!!).

Rob doesn't think that we have enough room in the car for all the stuff that we have, but when you have 3 females what do you expect? He should downsize to one pair of jeans, one sweater, and one sweatshirt - then we would have plenty of room!!!

I am feeling good and energized. However I did get cranky with the girls tonight. Sometimes it's very hard to pack with everyone at the same time, but we survived.

Someone asked me about the side effects on this chemo treatment. There was a 30% chance that I would lose my hair and I am not. I have the hardest day right after chemo, but by the third day I am pretty much back to normal. I should find out Dec 1st when the scan is and what the game plan is for after the IV chemo is done.

I better go. I am sure that even though Rob said we are leaving at 9:00am he will want to go sooner.

I will write when we get back
LOL!!

Do you really want to know???
Posted Dec 2, 2008 10:04pm

Hello my friends -
I hope you all had a nice holiday!!!

We have returned from the cold and snow to a balmy Kenosha; Sat. it was 41 degrees warmer here than up North. Thanksgiving week was very nice and VERY quiet. We did see 4-5 deer that were still alive and moving without the fear of hunters. Uncle Roger, Chuck, Aunt Diane, Uncle Howard and Nathan were with us over the holiday. We enjoyed lots of food (in fact I gained a pound - I was getting a bit concerned about my weight but all is well!) and great fires (in the fireplace) every night. I am not sure how many trees we went through. Raney and Becca decorated Christmas cookies that Diane made (should we mention that the lady gingerbread cookies were given chocolate chip boobies???). Raney and Becca decorated a gingerbread house. I tried to help but when Rob went to put the house together we discovered that what I thought was the roof really was the side of the house and Raney and Becca had decorated the roof pieces as the sides. Luckily the doors seemed to end in the right spot to make solar windows on the roof. I am teaching the kids to be green!!

I kidnapped my sister and made her stay another night in Kenosha before releasing her back to her crib in Rogers Park. I don't think she minded too much! She played Raney and Becca's new favorite game, Clue (thanks Uncle Roger!!!).

Saturday I played catch up with errands and grocery and Sunday we put up some of our Christmas decorations. When I have millions I might pay someone to do everything but the tree. I like to look at all the ornaments we have collected over the years.

Monday was the port placement and chemo day. Rob and I were up and out of the house by 5:45am. My sister-in-law was able to stay with Raney and Becca and get them to school on time (something that I am not always able to do, so that is quite an accomplishment).

The port placement went fine; no problems except my veins are starting to become difficult for IVs (three tries before the nurse was successful).

Then we went upstairs to check in for the chemo. I am not sure why the nurse did what she did, but she took off the surgical tape (this was covering the derma bond tape that was covering the incision that takes 7-14 days to fall off by itself and keeps the wound clean and dry) and replaced it with very strong tape. It took a long time for the chemo to get started. The nurse came in to pull the access to the port out and the tape took off the derma bond tape, so now I am exposed!!!

Of course, I was a bit freaked because I do not want another infection or pic line. After clearly stating that I didn't like the nurse's option of steri-strips, I was sent back down to the 4th floor for more derma bond tape. I think that Rob, Eileen and I got to the car around 4:30ish. Way too long if you ask me.

I, also, was to see the PA and she didn't show so I left. I had enough and I was tired and the nurse hurt me when she pulled off the tape.

Being frustrated with everything yesterday, I called Loyola Hospital today to make an appointment with another oncologist. I don't want to go somewhere where I am not given compassion and support beyond the right medicines. Maybe tomorrow when I call the doctor to voice my concerns I will decide that Northwestern is the right place, but there is nothing wrong with checking out other places. There are times in our lives where we leave relationships for various reasons, and this may be one of those times. Perhaps I need more than I can get at Northwestern. I am asking God to help me find the place I need to be at for support in all the areas that I need, not just the medicines!!!

On a better note, Becca is off to state this Saturday and I will be feeling great by then. Last night and today are the rough days. I don't eat much, and I feel like I could be sick at any time.

Regardless, I am thankful for being on this planet because tomorrow is a whole new start!!!

I better get to bed and see what types of dreams are waiting for me.

Have a wonderful day because, just like getting through winter makes spring that much sweeter, getting through the rough days makes the peaceful ones so much more of a blessing.

Many Hugs
P.S. And thanks for listening.

Happy Holidays
Posted Dec 14, 2008 7:53am

Hello my friends,
It's been awhile since I last chatted. As you know, this can be a busy time of the year trying to get ready for all the fun!!!

I won't back up to Dec. 3rd, but rest assured that I must be doing OK since I am shopping, decorating, and maintaining the house. One thing about the last couple of weeks - Becca was in a state meet for gymnastics and she placed in bar and beam!!! Afterwards we went to a town called New Glarus and had a nice afternoon - lunch, shopping, and we saw St. Nick (it was Dec 6th when we were there).

Fast forward to Thursday Dec 15th - a friend and I went to Evanston to stay the night (thanks Pam!!!) because of chemo on Friday. We did a little shopping (I really don't shop this much all year!!!) and then went out to dinner. Afterwards we worked on Christmas cards. On Friday morning we went out to breakfast and downtown for treatment. We walked the building before chemo to pick up the tests that I need to send to Loyola. Chemo went fine. I had my nurse who I used to see the last time around, which really helped because my white counts were a bit high. They are not sure why, so they drew more blood. (I can't believe I will have any left after all of this is said and done). But I was able to still be treated.

Afterwards we went shopping!! We met up with my dad to pick up the nativity scene that my family used growing up. I can't ruin the surprise, but I think everyone in the family will really like the way it is displayed - better than I had pictured!!! God works in mysterious ways.

When I was dropped off Rob was making soup and rum balls; Raney and Becca were out for the night. After dinner we watched a movie. It was nice (and quiet) just don't tell Raney and Becca.

Saturday we went and watched *The Nutcracker*. A friend of ours' daughter was in three roles (7th grader). It was really nice; a very Christmasy thing to do. However, I did go to bed at 7:30pm; I was tired. When Raney and Becca went to bed around 9:00pm, they crawled in with me. I think they sense when I am weak and not able to fend them off.

Now we are here today.

I haven't really talked about all the jewelry that I have been given throughout this journey but here is one to share:

A friend of mine's daughter - who is six - got a ring from the quarter machine that says LIVE. Hannah decorated a bag for me and drew a picture. The ring is blue with yellow writing and I have worn it since I got it.

I almost forgot to share the big news: I am being scanned on Monday –
tomorrow - bone and CAT scan. I will be shot with radioactive stuff and be
able to spin a strong web (which will come in handy with some of the ideas I
have for decorating) and then I have to drink VILE stuff. On the positive
side, I think I should have an answer and another game plan before the end
of the year. We are going to drink Champagne!!! Every day is a gift and this
season reminds me of all that God has blessed my family with. Yes, there are
some hardships we will remember this season (Sole being gone is one), but
God loves us and I am thankful for each day!!

Have a great day!!
Happy Holidays

The envelope, please!
Posted Dec 17, 2008 9:17pm

I am so tired, I should go to bed. But I think some of you are waiting with
baited breathe about the results.....
The scans went fine. There was a lot of poking me to give me radiation or
dye or to take my blood; nothing out of my new ordinary. It was a long day,
but then we came home to my sister cooking dinner - so nice!!

As you all know, what I truly wanted was a miracle of all miracles. I wanted
the doctors to see nothing and have no explanation except to say, "It's a
miracle!!" Well, I didn't get that, but I did get the next best thing - for the
most part - my lungs and spine responded very well to the chemo. I think
that they don't see anything on the lungs anymore and my bones are doing
well; the liver still needs some help. The cancer grew a bit, so I will be doing
some other chemo starting the 29th of Dec. I need to talk to the doctor
about the different options before we know the next step.

Yes, at first I was a bit disappointed because I want to start living like
other people and not have to go downtown every two weeks and be hooked up
to a machine, but as I think about it and talk to Rob, this is really pretty
good news. I could have heard the cancer grew in all three places and nothing
worked. Now that would have been really hard, so I am thankful (GOD) that
I did respond well and now we just need to get the liver under control. I

think that the problem was I kept picturing the liver as a red/brownish organ and it's not - maybe I won't be getting that MD degree after all. Now that I know the organ is pink, I will be getting my visualization better and the liver will respond.

I am waiting to schedule with the doctor and moving forward. And that is better than moving backwards.

Tomorrow I am talking with a nutritionist from UT that I sent my medical records to, and she sent me a report with foods and supplements to add to my team of destroyers of cancer cells. That is what I do every day with your help - KILL cancer cells. I have won some of the battles; now it's back to war to get the rest of the little bastards.

And on that note, Happy Holidays! Good cheer to you and your family!!! LOL

Merry Christmas!!
Posted Dec 21, 2008 10:27am

...and HAPPY NEW YEAR!!! I am gearing up for the new year to have even better news!!!

Rob and Raney are on their way to pick up Uncle Roger from O'Hare; it is like the North Pole out there. I have decided that penguins are cute but crazy! Have you watched *The March of the Penguins*? I don't want to come back as a penguin.

I ventured out to church this morning and the deacon was talking about how the best gift is the gift of ourselves, but it is also the hardest gift to give. So, I want to thank you all again for taking time to remember me, Rob, and the girls as this journey is upon us for a LONG time (that is what God and I talk about every night). Life gets crazy and time flies, but I still receive cards, messages on the blogs, calls, and (most importantly) prayers.

Tomorrow we are heading downtown to freeze and to talk to the doctor about what options are ahead of me. The PA did mention something about a clinical trial so maybe I will be part of something big!!! I know that my body does respond well to medicine; now I just need something that works with the PINK liver (I never should have fallen asleep in science).

As Christmas approaches I pray to God to help me remember Christmas is not about the cleanest house, the best decorations, or even the juiciest turkey, but all the love we share, the memories we make, and the best grab bag gift!!! (And I pray that Rob remembers this as well - so please send light his way too!!!!!!!)

One more note and then I have to clean and get the decorations up and pluck the turkey.

Please pray for Ceci, Angi, and Andrea as they face their first Christmas without their mom, Sole.

We miss you Sole, and hope you have plenty of peace in Heaven!!
LOL

Posted Dec 25, 2008 10:38pm

I still have a couple of hours before I am late with the holiday cheers!!!

Rob and I met with the doctor on Monday. She isn't concerned with the cancer in the bone. She said the organs are much more important. The lungs had small spots before and she was happy they were gone, but the liver gives her the most concern because the spots there grew. But never fear - underdog is here! Not really. The doctor said that I have a lot of good liver left; God gives us more then we need.

Ok, everyone get your medical books! I signed up for the trial which starts Monday Dec 29th. I am not sure what group I am going to be in, but the chemos are either Ixabepilone plus Capecitadine, or Docetaxel plus Capecitadine. Ixabepilone and Docetaxel are IV chemos the other one, Capecitadine, is a pill. I will take the IV and then 2 weeks of the pill form. (Are you confused, yet? There will be a test on Monday). Two out of the three groups take 3 hours to get the chemo and the last group is an hour.

I have rules with this study so I have to get organized (not sure about that rule). I have to ALWAYS carry the clinical study alert card with me (so that way no other medicines can be administered and mess up my part of the study); I have to keep a dosing diary; and I have to complain about every nook and cranny - that will make Rob very happy (he would like me to become a complainer as he doesn't trust that I tell him the truth when I don't feel well.) I just don't think rules and chemo are the best combo...

Shall we talk about the side effects? So much fun!
In about nine weeks - if I handle the meds well - I get to be bald again. Now the biggest problem with this is, I just purchased a gallon of shampoo/conditioner that the nutritionist recommended. Thank God that Raney and Becca have long hair. Honestly, I am not looking forward to being bald again, but at least winter should be over (I hope; it is not looking too promising in Kenosha but the days are getting longer!!!!).

Fatigue – OK, I wouldn't mind a break from this side effect but I have had this since Raney was born.

Low white counts means more shots...and then many, many more.

We have been partying since Dec. 23rd - starting with Rob's godson, Charlie, and his parents; then Christmas Eve with Rob's cousins; then Christmas with my side of the family; and then on Dec 26th Rob's sister and her family will be ready to party some more.

Last night we went to midnight mass at 11:00pm. It was very nice. Both girls slept for about a half hour. As Becca was sleeping, I was playing with her hair. My new fetish: hair. I tried to do some visualization with my eyes closed, but Rob thought I was falling asleep, so he kept poking me to see if I needed to go home.

When we got home and the girls went to bed, "Santa" filled the stockings and thought everything was good and went to bed with sugar plums and dancing fairies and partridges jiggling all the way home. Then the morning happened...

155

Santa put the wrong names on two gifts (Santa did this last year as well) and the stockings that were hung so carefully had three scratch-off lottery tickets and that was it -no nail polish or bubble baths. I think Santa is getting fired this year. I hope the new Santa enjoys wrapping everything and getting it all right. (I have only messed up on my chemo years, but since I will be on some type of chemo for the rest of my life, maybe the red coat should be hung out to dry.)

All is calm on the western front. We had a wonderful Christmas; the turkey was juicy, the wine had enough breath to taste great, and plenty of sweets to satisfy 21 people plus 5 kids. Sole was sadly missed, and the girls are struggling, so prayers are still needed for them.

I was telling someone tonight that I wouldn't choose this journey, nor would any family member choose this for me, but I look for the roses along the path. Sometimes they are very hard to find, but they are always there. I sometimes need the help of my family and friends to see the beauty in all this; and I have family and friends that are always walking by my side showing me the many gifts of cancer.

As odd as it seems, the gifts truly are there.

Gifts of:
a new appreciation for life
slowing down
less housework
no shoveling
no raking leaves
meals delivered

I know that God has me surrounded by Angels and they are called my family and friends.

I think I need to go to bed because I am no longer sure I am making any sense.

I hope all of you had a blessed Christmas and that the last week of 2008 is a magical one.

There is still time to do this year's resolution - except for maybe organizing the front hall closet, just keep that one on the list for next year.
Good night and sweet dreams (unless you ate too many sweets, just have a nice dream then).

Inquiring minds want to know...
Posted Jan 1, 2009 3:42pm

I am a bit behind in letting you all know what has happened since Rob and I spoke with the doctor.

I may have told you that I am in the clinical trial. I would have been put on the same chemo regardless, but this gets me watched much more closely. The next time I am scanned, they will measure more spots & I will see either the PA or the doctor at every visit.

After waiting a week from Dec 22 to Dec 29, I finally have an answer, but before we get to that, I hope all of you had a wonderful Christmas/New Year's break. We got an extra day due to 12-13 inches of snow dumped on us Dec 19th, but that didn't stop Becca's brownie troop from caroling that night (just like the mailmen).
We celebrated a first b-day (and I went to a 40th b-day party later that day). I just love birthdays, and I hope to have a LARGE number more.
Roger (brother-in-law) came into town for fun and parties for the week. This is just a quick recap, but it was a wonderful week full of family and friends.
Raney and Becca could have used many more hours of sleep since we are back to the routine in three days (it will be just like the first week of school trying to get back into the swing of things).
Rob did major cooking on the 23, 24, 25, 26, and then he was able to take a break.
Santa was kind to all of us and I hope none of you got coal in your stocking! Everything was perfect except for Santa mismarking a couple of presents, and forgetting to stuff Raney and Becca's stockings. (Santa and chemo do not mix.) But now I have bribery gifts for 2010!!!!

157

On Monday the 29th we went to Chicago to get the new chemo and my new diary. How exciting – even gifts from the doctors this season!!!

My brother took the girls to Navy Pier and Rob and I went to the 21st Floor. I was called back quickly (maybe a perk of being in a trial? Remember there is a rose hidden everywhere!). My numbers were great - I even had the blood tests done that the nutritionist wanted. My sister and brother-in-law surprised us with a hotel room at the same Marriot that they were staying at (close to the hospital if anything were to happen - one of the worst side effects is that I could stop breathing, but I get the impression that the doctors know how to get my breathing back).

Rob and I waited in the waiting area to be told that I need to be clean for four weeks. I have to be off the last chemo for 4 weeks before they can start anything new with me. That piece of information was not told to us, so we called Jimee and had him and the girls meet us for lunch at The Drake (Rob likes their bookbinder soup, aka turtle soup, not my favorite). Then we went to the American Girl store and made our way back to the hotel. We went out to dinner with some of the family and then back to the hotel where the kids and Aidan swam until 10ish. The next day we took the girls back to Navy Pier and had lunch at the Billy Goat grill. It was like being on a surprise vacation – and it would have been cheaper to get chemo!!!! (But I prefer a surprise vacation.) I weighed myself at the work out and I think I maintained my weight!!!

The new chemo date is Jan 16th; it's every three weeks and after 3 cycles I will be re-scanned and bald again. As Raney states, I am ready to be bald because she had the hat party and we have lots of things for my head. At least I had hair for this winter!! It's not so much being bald as the grow out didn't do much for me because of the curls - they drove me nuts!!

We rang in the New Year with some friends and now I am ready for a nap!!! We all were up past midnight.

And now I need to reflect on 2009 to see what I might resolve to do this year...
Keep working on inner peace.
Heal!!!!!!!!!

Make it a rocking year!!!
I am going to work on my pictures more.
Create a company that grows leaps and bounds.
With all the prayers that God hears on my account, I think I have a good chance to shock the doctors in 13-14 weeks when I get rescanned. I will have lots of prayers said, will be eating better, and I am very clear of what I ask from God. So I am ready for the next stage...

Until I chat again
HAPPY NEW YEAR!!!

Me and my shadow
Posted Jan 1, 2009 10:25pm

This won't be long, I promise. I should be going to bed but I still don't understand this journey.

I went to see *Marley and Me*, a very cute movie. When I got home, I had to walk my Marley Jr. (who is about 12 pounds so her destruction is not nearly as bad as the movie dog) and the weather is cold, but the night is so clear - lots of stars in Kenosha. I am feeling GREAT!!! I really feel great. And I have doctors telling me otherwise. I am just confused. I am TRUELY grateful for feeling good; I don't want to feel like the paper says about me, but I have this shadow over me - it never leaves me anymore. I don't like that. It's not a shadow that takes away my ability to enjoy life, in fact it helps me appreciate things so much more, but I want it gone. It can turn on me at anytime, and I don't like that feeling.

On that note, I am going to bed. No worries, my shadow doesn't keep me up or stop me from doing what I do; it is not a weight, it is just a presence.

Another Change in the plans
Posted Jan 8, 2009 9:24pm

It is Thursday, about 9:00 p.m., and Patty asked me to add this update because Rob needs the internet. Today is Becca's 9th birthday and the family had a nice birthday dinner. Before they left, Patty was called and was told that she needs to see the doctor at 8:30 tomorrow morning. She then goes for an EKG and she finds out which clinical study she will be put in.

Because Patty and Rob need to leave at 6:00 a.m., the girls are staying at a friend's house. Carrie is making a birthday cake, picking up a game and watching the dog; Becca is so excited.

We will let you know what is going on after Patty finds out what is going on

Jimee

Planes, trains and automobiles
Posted Jan 9, 2009 2:37pm

Taxotere is the winner.

Patty began her journey to Chicago in the snow, with Rob taking his car in for repairs. The plan was for Patty to follow Rob to the dealer and then drive in together. Mother Nature had different plans. As usual, the plans fell off the track and Patty stopped in Evanston to park at my friend's condo, taking the train from there. Rob stopped in Lake Bluff and took the train in. Both will be taking the train to Lake Bluff and I will get their car for them.

The taxotere is the 1 hour intravenous chemo, rather than the 3 hours, every three weeks. 2x per day, for 14 days, Patty needs to take 3 pills. That is 6 pills a day. She is required to keep track of this while dealing with chemo brain. Let's see how long that lasts.

Patty is behind me and is joking, so her spirits are good. Waiting for hours makes her a little testy, and Rob a little more testy.

Some good news: Patty gained 2lbs. Her new eating plan must be working. She remembers the carbs.

Patty will be updating with her good cheer soon.

Jimee

I'm back
Posted Jan 16, 2009 10:47pm

Sorry it has been awhile, but it took awhile to recover from my field trip to Hell and back and now I am freezing my ASS off here in Kenosha (just like my body hot flashes and then cold - no middle ground here; a whopping -4 at the moment).

OK, shall we recap? Chemo a week ago, Becca's b-day party Sat, and then we went and saw *Grease* ("is the word"...brought back some good memories), then a half a week of school. Raney and Becca had no school. Didn't they just stay home 2 weeks for Christmas? I might have chemo brain, but I swear I think I am seeing a little too much of them these days. And Monday is a half day (they get out at 11:00am) Why do I even bother taking them?

Rob was out of town for the fun "cold" days of no school, but my sister-in-law picked the little straw and stayed with us for a couple of days. We played Life and had a couple of fires (in the fireplace). She made me breakfast and helped get the kids ready for bed. And because of no school, we were able to sleep in until 9:00am!!! That was very nice because I was still tired from the chemo day. I think the train is starting to sound like a good option again. I don't think there will be anymore passing out in my life. I tried it and it is not fun; gets me too many days/nights in the hospital. I promise to behave. I still have my ten ride punch card that is only good for a year.

I went to Loyola for a second opinion and the doctor said that the treatment Northwestern has me on is very aggressive. I think the only difference is that she would try me on a hormonal treatment instead of chemo right now.

161

I guess my doctor had written some notes about her decision of putting me on chemo, and I think if I had the choice I would have chosen the chemo, at least one more time. I seem to respond to chemo, and I handle it OK. At least for now. I am getting more tired, but I am hoping these two extra sleep-in days will help me out. It was good to get a second opinion for peace of mind, but I won't be changing to Loyola.

I forgot to share with you that I am on chemo pills for two weeks and then a week off. The side effects can be quite gruesome with what can happen to my hands and feet. And, I kid you not; it states that no housework should be done. I am off the hook for doing housework because of medical reasons!!!! I might learn to love Xeloda!! I am kidding, I would rather do housework than be on these pills forever, but while I am on them I will just have to follow the rules!!! I am not to cause any friction to my hands. I am also not supposed to wear gloves while doing dishes so that is off my list because I won't wash dishes without gloves. And I am supposed to stay out of the sun - not a hard one to follow with -30 wind chill.

I remember telling someone that I wanted to get to the point where I get to take a pill and not have to go downtown all the time. I forgot to state that I wanted to stop taking the IV form of chemo. Now I get to do both so I need to learn that when asking for something, I need to be a bit clearer. Now when I tell God that I want to stay on Earth I state 'for many earthly years' since I am not sure how Heaven time works versus our time. Clarity is a good thing. But I am hoping God gives people with chemo brain a little leeway.

At the moment I am not having any problems with the new chemo. I am tired (and probably should be in bed) but I think that is a result of the holidays still. I do have to watch for this hand/foot problem - blistering and discoloration of the appendages. I just lost a thought that I am sure was a gut buster - sorry I am not able to make you laugh today. Now I remember, they sent me UDDER CREAM - used on real cows. I am not sure how I feel about this. I was given two of them, but at least if I don't use them, Raney and Becca don't have to fight over Udder cream. I am not sure how I would handle that fight.

We went and saw *Mall Cop* tonight. I laughed a few times. It was a lot better than I thought it would be. Tomorrow a friend is making us Thai food. And then a family b-day party for the Jan b-days (Sharon, Becca, & Katy) (Uncle Frank and Eddie, we will sing even though we are in two different places).

I just love b-days. I am not sure if I have always felt this way or just since Kevin left us. Birthdays are full of life; plus, who doesn't like cake, pizza and presents?? Maybe I should treat every day as a birthday because just like it is 5:00pm somewhere, it is someone's b-day.

I think it is time to say good-night. I am hanging in there and sometimes it is by a thread. I don't think Becca is going to give me the Best mommy award quite yet, but I am trying. Sometimes it is hard, but the gifts of life keep me going - and you all are the gifts of my life. Thanks again for your prayers, thoughts, food, books, CDs, cleanings, blankets, wines, company, babysitting and more. I will never be able to thank you properly so I am going to let God do that when you reach the pearly gates. Just know I don't take you for granted.

Before the end of the month and the New Year's resolution idea seems too late to start, try telling someone new how important they are to you. Let's get the ripple of kindness going for 2009. This world needs lots of kind words to heal. Let's see if we can make a ripple!!

Sweet dreams and have fun!!
Love to all

Hi there
Posted Jan 26, 2009 11:48am

Yes, I know that it has been a while since I last spoke to you, but rest assured, I am feeling great. The biggest side effect that I have since the beginning of the #3 chemo round (and three times is a charm, so I am expecting only the greatest of great this time around) is the hand syndrome - it dries out your hands worse than any winter wind. But I went to Reiki and I walked out with my arms tingling and my hands have been better ever since. I am still putting on the lotion, but the redness is 90% gone. Another thing about Reiki is they talk about the charkas and their colors (this is the energy map of our bodies). I now have a billion plus rainbows in my body

163

because every cell is a rainbow. I told my sister that if an autopsy was done on my body, all they would see are rainbows under the microscope (not that I want an autopsy).

On Jan 17 Rob, the girls and I went to a friend's house who cooks Thai food. One of his curry dishes was very SPICY (and I used to do spicy a lot better than I am able to do now), but the food was fabulous and we had so much fun. Raney ate 5 platefuls and I think Becca ate about 4. Terry, the chef, was amazed at what they could eat. (It almost seemed like I don't feed them!) The kids were sent downstairs and the adults stayed upstairs dancing, singing and sharing stories. We laughed and ate and ate and laughed.

On Jan 18 my sister had her b-day and we went to Larry and Sharon's party room to celebrate the Jan b-days (Sharon, Katy and Becca). Larry made SPICY chili, a salad and, of course, there was a big birthday cake. As you know, we have been trying to get together monthly as a family, so this was our monthly silly Sunday. Katy bought Becca this game called Build a Sentence. You have to build a sentence in two minutes out of 10 cards (these are pentagon shaped and have different tenses of the same word). Sounds easy, but it is so not!!! By the end of the party, we were all sitting around playing (and at this point we decided to have teams to help each other out) or being judges to determine if the sentence passed. We laughed and argued with each other, but the main judge would not budge. She was one tough cookie (Hi Sue!!). Katy and I hold the record for the most points for one sentence (80!!). Chemo Brains Rule!!!

When I was getting ready for bed and I brushing my teeth, my mouth started to be on fire again and I thought, I am in trouble now! Then I saw I had put on the wrong toothpaste. My poor tongue had no breaks from the spicy that weekend.

Monday I woke up feeling great! Laughter is what is needed every day. That really is the best medicine; the kind of laughing when you think your gut is going to explode.
The rest of the week went normal: getting up for school, running out the door with breakfast in hand, and trying to stay warm as I walked the dog. I am working on building up my sister's business. I want to create a career that I am able to do from my house.

The other thing is I signed up for a course at the University of WI-Parkside (I am going back to school!) on writing a book. The person teaching is Brian Barnes and I am hoping he is related to Barnes and Noble. I am moving forward with writing a book! I have had many comments about that and I am ready. 2009 is a year of ACTION and I am so ready to be active in many ways. My ideas need to become *more*...and I have lots of them. I am not sure if they will work, but I will never know if they stay ideas.

There is another challenge for all of us: take an idea and put an action to it this year.

This weekend was very quiet. The kids and I saw *Hotel for Dogs*. I thought it was good. Sunday we hung out with Aidan and Larry. We went out for dinner with Jimee and Katy for Becca's b-day dinner - all you can eat sushi (Becca's favorite food). That is all I am saying on that dinner, but let me tell you that is the way to eat sushi - with my kids!!!
(I am not sure we will be seated the next time we go!)

Today, the children don't have school, so one went outside to hammer fire wood together and I am not sure what the other one is doing. I think I might need to go locate her. But it is quiet so I might wait for the screams...
Keep warm if you are somewhere over the rainbow and its cold.

Have a great day and we will chat soon-

P.S. My writing class starts next Monday for 4 classes.

Hugs and Smiles

P.P.S. I think that my hair is starting to fall out. I had some strands on the pillow and in the sink. I am not sure if it is normal hair fallout or if it is chemo hair fallout. (But I don't usually have as many strands on the pillow case and sink as I did today.) All I have to say about this round of getting bald is I am so happy that I didn't get my hair highlighted. See good in everything!!!!!

Hello everyone,
I am in need of a haircut as I am now waking up to strands like I have never seen before on my pillow. And, as my loving husband said, I looked better bald then how my hair looks now. The love flows in this household!!!! (His hamburger was a bit more burnt than usual – ha, ha).

Lori is coming over in about an hour to give me my second (and last) balding haircut. I don't mind the baldness as much as the growing out phase. Here I am a little over a year of growing back, back at the length I wear my hair, and now it's got to go.

Maybe I will embrace the baldness more so when it gets warm, though I am beginning to wonder about that here in WI! More fun, more action, all in 2009!!!! Maybe this Halloween I will be Fester!!!!

I have to get ready for the big haircut

talk to you soon,
hugs and smiles.

Posted Jan 30, 2009 9:19pm

I feel 100%, except I learned that you don't take steroids at night. It kept me up past midnight. I thought all steroids did was help gain muscles - I must have slept through that drug lesson.

I had two of my sisters with me today, and we had a wonderful time. In fact, I didn't really pay attention to the drugs dripping into my body. I put Katy to work making baby shower cards and Eileen massaging my feet. What more does one need? Oh, I remember, Katy walking 158 feet to get lunch!!!

Afterwards we went to a store called Lush (high end soaps and lotions). My hands are reacting to the chemo pills. The employee gave us all hand massages. It was Heaven on earth.

My neighbor made us dinner tonight and they stayed and ate with us so the whole day was very pleasant. A perfect chemo day; and after the last time of 14 hours of HELL this is what the doctor ordered.

Oh, and the doctor said no to skiing because if I were to break something, my treatments would have to stop. I can still have a great time watching - it is just that my kids wanted me to ski, so I had to ask.

I just wanted to get in a quick update. I am getting tired and I just might have to end this perfect day.

I wish you all happy dreams filled with warm breezes and pina coladas (for those 21 and over).

hugs and smiles!!!

Posted Feb 2, 2009 8:44am

Today is the big day: I start my life as a writer and class is at 7:00pm. (I just hope that I can stay up for the big event!!)

Today started out rough; I am not sure how much I slept last night and my calves are sore. I feel like a cold is coming on and food isn't tasting very good; I forgot about that side effect (and that is a real bummer).

That is all the complaining I am going to do because regardless of what the groundhog saw today winter will soon be put away for awhile!!!! I just keep imagining the warm breeze on my face and I know there are better days ahead. I am not worried about a slow day in the least. I might even get a nap in!!!

Enjoy the BIG day. I love Groundhog Day!!!

Until I write again
Smile and Hugs to all

Epilogue

Wow!! Time flies when I am having fun. It's been awhile since I have last blogged for my friends, so let's catch up.

I was told on December 2, 2010 that the spots on the liver had grown and that I was going to be back on chemo. This was after being off chemo for 11 beautiful months. I had hair and energy back. My doctor was surprised that I was off chemo for that long. She had told me that I would be on chemo for the rest of my life, with taking breaks. I believed with all my heart that I was not ever going to be on chemo ever again. With this news, I went to a very dark place during the weekend. I was fighting with my family. I told my sister," I can't do this anymore. I give up."

Luckily, I was only there for the weekend. This is not an easy journey. And sometimes the journey gets really rocky for me and I do just want to jump in the river and have it be over. I then remember that I am not alone and that is why I can get up off the floor and move forward. Never underestimate your importance to me—even if it is just a message on carepages, a quick email, or a text (now). Without you and the grace of God, I wouldn't be here.

Yesterday, I took Raney for her 13th year physical—she passed. While we were driving home, I remembered how at the beginning of this journey I thought that I wouldn't be here for these days. I no longer have those thoughts. The time of worry is over. I am now doing what I do best and what I do best is LOL: Lots of Love; Laughing out Loud; Living out Loud!

PS: I was scanned today—"Your scans are much approved. Your liver is much better. Everything looks great. I'm very happy with the way things are looking." -Dr. Kaklamina

I am going to continue chemo though so that I can get the rest of the rat bastards out of me.

Until then...

Lol, Patty

Acknowledgements

First I would like to acknowledge Theresa Serpe for doing the first edit on this book and Colleen Kappeler for doing the final edit. Without their input I would still be working on 'then' and 'than'! Thanks also to Colleen Kappeler for doing the book layout for her masters' class.

Next I would like to thank my talented sister Katy Dunn for the cover layout, my sweet sister-in-law Kristin Dunn for the cover design, and my dear friend Wendi Hawkins for taking the photo which graces the cover. You ladies rock!

I also want to thank my brother Jimee Dunn for his humor and ability to keep me posted in a timely fashion when I was unable to do so.

I want to thank my dear friend Carrie Greskowviak for organizing meals for us for after my chemo – and of course I want to thank all the families who contributed meals! We ate them all. (My weight is proof!)

I want to thank Dr. Virginia Kaklamani and Gina Uthe, PA, as well as all the staff at Northwestern. I pray for a cure in our lifetime. And a special thanks to Harmony Hill for offering a place of solace and community for cancer patients.

And finally a shout out to www.carepages.com, a place where I blogged my hopes, fears and progress for my community to read and respond. Without carepages I wouldn't have known the amount of support and love out there for me.

Made in the USA
Charleston, SC
22 August 2011